Mental Health i

This book provides a comprehensive overview of mental health in rural America, with the goal of fostering urgently needed research and honest conversations about providing accessible, culturally competent mental health care to rural populations. Grounding the work is an explanation of the history and structure of rural mental health care, the culture of rural living among diverse groups, and the crucial "A's" and "S": accountability, accessibility, acceptability, affordability, and stigma. The book then examines poverty, disaster mental health, ethics in rural mental health, and school counseling. It ends with practical information and treatments for two of the most common problems, suicide and substance abuse, and a brief exploration of collaborative possibilities in rural mental health care.

Ellen Greene Stewart, MA, ATR-BC, LCAT, is a New York state-licensed, board-certified creative arts therapist who has been in private practice in rural upstate New York for more than 15 years. She is the author of two previous books, *Kaleidoscope* and *Superheroes Unmasked*, and numerous peer reviewed articles, and has worked with a wide variety of populations. She can be reached at peacebaby@catskill.net.

Mental Health in Rural America
A Field Guide

Ellen Greene Stewart

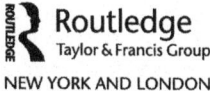

NEW YORK AND LONDON

First published 2018
by Routledge
711 Third Avenue, New York, NY 10017

and by Routledge
2 Park Square, Milton Park, Abingdon, Oxon, OX14 4RN

Routledge is an imprint of the Taylor & Francis Group, an informa business

© 2018 Ellen Greene Stewart

The right of Ellen Greene Stewart to be identified as author of this work has been asserted by her in accordance with sections 77 and 78 of the Copyright, Designs and Patents Act 1988.

All rights reserved. No part of this book may be reprinted or reproduced or utilised in any form or by any electronic, mechanical, or other means, now known or hereafter invented, including photocopying and recording, or in any information storage or retrieval system, without permission in writing from the publishers.

Trademark notice: Product or corporate names may be trademarks or registered trademarks, and are used only for identification and explanation without intent to infringe.

Library of Congress Cataloging-in-Publication Data
Names: Stewart, Ellen Greene, author.
Title: Mental health in rural America : a field guide/Ellen Greene Stewart.
Description: New York : Routledge, 2018. | Includes bibliographical references and index.
Identifiers: LCCN 2017049920 | ISBN 9781138729452 (hbk : alk. paper) | ISBN 9781138729469 (pbk : alk. paper) | ISBN 9781315189857 (ebk)
Subjects: LCSH: Rural mental health services—United States.
Classification: LCC RA790.6. S74 2018 | DDC 362.20973—dc23
LC record available at https://lccn.loc.gov/2017049920

ISBN: 978-1-138-72945-2 (hbk)
ISBN: 978-1-138-72946-9 (pbk)
ISBN: 978-1-315-18985-7 (ebk)

Typeset in Galliard
by Apex CoVantage, LLC

This book is dedicated to my dad, Kenneth A. Greene, the best dad and a truly self-made man whose love of nature led him from the Bronx to the Catskill Mountains. In doing this, he led me to the rural life I love. He never lost sight of his values, led by example, taught me to do the right thing and make a difference. I am grateful to have inherited some of his strengths, especially his love of learning.

Contents

About the Author xii
Acknowledgments xiii
Preface: Rural America—Bucolic and Beleaguered xiv
Introduction: Rural Matters—Life in a Hamlet xvi

1 **What Defines Rural and Frontier, and Why Are They Important?** 1
   Formal and Informal Definitions 1
   Defining Rural and Frontier 2
   Rural Matters: YOU ARE HERE 4
   A Few Words on the Terms Behavioral Health and Mental Health 5
   What Does a Rural Mental Health Professional Look Like? 5
   References 6

2 **Rural Mental Health Policy and Parity** 8
   History of Rural Mental Health 8
   A Timeline of Mental Health in Rural America 8
   The Mental Health Parity Act of 2008 and the Difficulties in Enforcing Parity 18
   The Affordable Care Act (ACA) 19
   Implications of the Affordable Care Act 20
   The Cures Act of 2016 22
   The Implications of Medicaid Redesign 23
   What Does Rural Mental Health Look Like Now? 24
   References 25

3 **Obstacles to Treatment—The Four "A's" and an "S": Accessibility, Availability, Acceptability, Affordability, and Stigma** 28
   What Are the Four A's, Their Implications, and Epidemiology? 28
   Accessibility 29
   Availability 30

Rural Mental Health Realities 32
Acceptability 32
Affordability 34
The "S" Word: Stigma—Its Causes and Implications
   in Rural Areas 38
Rural Matters: The Memorial Day Parade 40
References 41

4 The Structure of Rural Mental Health Care: State, County, Town, Village 44
The Structure of Local Governments 44
The Community Services Board (CSB) 45
Community Mental Health Centers (CMHC) 46
References 46

5 Understanding the Culture of Rural Living 48
Families 49
Men 49
Women 50
Infants and Children 51
Rural Matters: Alone on a Hilltop 53
Adolescents 55
The Elderly 56
Indigenous Populations: American Indians and Alaska Natives 57
Veterans—Visible and Invisible Injuries 59
Refugees and Undocumented Immigrants 60
Migrant Workers 61
Victims of Domestic Violence (DV) 62
Incarcerated Populations and Sex Offenders 64
Bringing Home the Bacon ... or Not: The Persistence of Poverty 66
Weapons Ownership 67
The LGBTQ Population 68
Disabled Individuals 70
   Physically Disabled Individuals 70
   Intellectually Disabled Individuals 70
The Homeless 71
Rural Matters: The First Day of Spring 73
References 74

6 Agricultural Roots of Rurality 77
The Farm Crisis 77
The Farm Bill 81

Famous Farming Quotes 83
Key Facts on Farming in the United States 84
The Critical Need for Affordable Insurance 85
Rural Matters: The Farm Crisis Hits Home 85
References 88

7 Disaster Mental Health — 90
Natural Disasters 91
Man-Made Disasters 95
References 96

8 Poverty — 97
Poverty Is a Constant in Rural Life 97
Needs Assessments in Rural Areas 99
Rural Matters: What Defines Life? 100
References 102

9 Types of Mental Health Practitioners and Their Scopes of Practice — 104
What Is "Scope of Practice"? 105
Psychiatrists 108
Psychologists 108
Psychiatric Nurse Practitioners 109
Licensed Mental Health Counselors or Licensed Marriage and Family Therapists 110
Licensed Clinical Social Workers 110
Mobile Crisis Teams and Crisis Respite 111
Art Therapists, Music, Dance/Movement, and Drama Therapy 112
Peer Advocates and Other Paraprofessionals 113
Pastoral Counselors 115
Primary Care Physicians (PCPs)—Issues With Providing Psychotropic Medications 115
Itinerant Counseling/Outreach 115
Training for Rural Work 116
References 117

10 Treatment Philosophies and Models — 120
The Flavor of the Year: Beyond CBT for All 120
Ecopsychology 121
The Sanctuary Model 122
Community Psychology 123

Trauma-Informed Therapy 124
The Public Health Approach 124
References 126

11 Issues in Rural Practice   127
Ethics in Rural Mental Health 127
Other Issues in Rural Mental Health 129
References 132

12 The Three "R's" of Schools in Rural Areas: Reassurance, Responsibility, and Resolution   136
Adverse Childhood Experiences (ACEs) and Their Lingering Effects 139
The President's New Freedom Commission's Recommendations for Children 140
References 141

13 Substance Abuse in Rural Areas   143
Prevalence, Causes, and Risk Factors 143
Alcohol 145
The Opioid Epidemic 146
The Morphine Element 148
Treatment Methods 149
Rural Matters: Hungry to Be Full 150
Rural Matters: Hump of the Moon 151
References 153

14 Suicide in Rural Areas   156
Prevalence, Causes, and Risk Factors 156
Shocking Statistics About Suicide in America 157
Risk Factors and Prevention Strategies for Suicide 158
Treatment for Suicidal Individuals 159
Rural Matters: The Last Straw 161
References 162

15 A Day in the Life of a Rural Mental Health Practitioner   165
Occupational Hazards 165
My Ride to Work 167
My Decision to Enter Private Practice 168
Rural Matters: A Paper Person 170
References 171

16 **The Rural Economy in Transition**   174
    Redefining Livelihood 174
    References 180

17 **Technological Innovations in Rural Mental Health Services**   182
    Telepsychology 182
    Challenges in Telepsychology 184
    References 186

18 **Looking Forward: Collaborative Possibilities**   188
    A Word About Funding and Developing Promising Practices 197
    Quotes on the Nation's Heartland 199
    References 199

    Mental Health Organizations   202
    Recommended Reading   214
    Index   215

About the Author

Ellen Greene Stewart, MA, ATR-BC, LCAT, is a board certified, licensed art therapist/counselor in who has been in private practice in rural upstate New York for the past 16 years. Ms. Stewart has an MA in Counseling Psychology from Goddard College. She is the author of two previous books—*Kaleidoscope* (Magnolia Street, 2006) is about the uses of art therapy with people with dementia, and *Superheroes Unmasked* is an original curriculum teaching grade school children emotional literacy skills such as self-esteem, team building, leadership training, and the psychology of bullying.

In addition to her previous books, she has written many journal articles and book and video reviews for peer reviewed journals.

She lives on a self-described "farmlet" in rural upstate New York with her husband, daughter, sheepdog, and an assortment of rescued rabbits and chickens. She can be reached at peacebaby@catskill.net.

Acknowledgments

Thanks to the staff at Routledge for recognizing the need for this book and helping bring it to life, Sharon Israel Cucinotta, Ev Ellsworth, Ann Epner, Doug Elston, Lilly Golden, Cindy Heaney, Maxine Borowsky Junge, Robbie Martin, Sarah Nies, William Rendler, Rina Riba, Arnie and Carol Schwartz, Bob and Lacey Stewart, Anique Taylor.

Author's Note: In this fast changing age of information, the facts, as written within this book, were known to be true at the time of publication.

> *We stand on the doorstep to make momentous progress in advancing the cause of this new civil rights struggle started by the work of President Kennedy over 50 years ago . . .* **We are in a race for inner space.**
>
> —Patrick Kennedy

Preface
Rural America—Bucolic and Beleaguered

This book answers the question: how does 25% of the population in the United States, residing on more than 90% of our land mass, get the mental health help they need? It also points out the countless issues practitioners need to be aware of in order to consider themselves culturally competent in "rurality." This is the book I sought but was unable to find when I first wanted to know more about mental health in rural America.

Accessibility, availability, acceptability, affordability, and stigma are the largest barriers to rural residents getting the mental health services they need. Many are the issues rural residents face. Those issues are not all particular to rurality but are more prevalent in rural areas than urban areas, making it harder to find services. There are several important ethical considerations rural practitioners face that differ from those of urban practitioners. Licensing and insurance laws are huge obstacles for some practitioners who want to practice in rural areas. Some promising solutions are on the horizon, but their implementation is slow, and they bring with them new issues.

My hope is that this book will heighten awareness about rural mental health and rural life in general that will ultimately help shift the paradigm of urban-oriented thinking to a more balanced viewpoint. In doing so I hope it will bring rural issues to the forefront. Urbanormativity is the general view of urban as "normal" and rural as second-rate, unimportant, and even in many ways, forgotten. It is in an urbancentric society we find ourselves shouting to have our rural voices heard.

It is my hope that this book will enhance the understanding of the changes that have historically taken place and those that are currently taking place in rural America, I also hope that it will contribute to a better understanding by rural residents themselves, by the general public, and by planners, developers, educators, community leaders, politicians, physicians, and mental health practitioners. I hope that it will stimulate many urgently needed research projects on the concerns discussed in this book, and stimulate open, honest conversations that seek to find solutions to these important issues. We need to join together to effect the positive changes needed in rural America in order to make rural life more livable. Whatever benefits rural life will ultimately benefit urban life, as we are two parts of a whole.

I chose this subject for intellectual reasons, but more importantly because the topic is my life day in and day out. I have spent so much time feeling frustrated about the lack of mental health resources in rural areas, both as a consumer and as a practitioner, and feeling frustrated in finding employment in this rural area I have chosen to call home. My frustration reached the point that I was spending all my energy on worrying about what I will do next to make a living, that I am grateful to be able to just put all that energy to use doing what I love—helping those who want help in my adopted home. I hope that this book will bring these rural issues to the forefront so that the conversation will continue yielding positive solutions. That way everyone wins.

Introduction
Rural Matters—Life in a Hamlet

When the noon whistle blows, we hear it everywhere. When the fire siren rings, the chances are that I know whoever is having an emergency, or I know their family. I live in the kind of town where everyone knows your name. It's the kind of town where it is considered rude not to wave to an oncoming car. It is home to 2,502 people. It is expected that we live and let live in order not to be slandered by the gossip. When I walk my dog, everyone greets us both by name. Here, even people who don't get along come to each other's aid in the face of adversity.

It is the kind of town where weather levels the playing field. It's the land of frost heaves and ice jams, where temperatures race to both ends of the spectrum. But there are those glowing Catskill days where the mild temperatures and clear blue skies make us feel we haven't a care in the world. That's what we live for.

This is a town without a traffic light, and where many roads remain dirt. Where else can you live where you know and check on each other's children and parents, and when a stray dog enters your yard, you know who to call to retrieve him. Where else can you know almost everyone in the Memorial Day parade as the progression marches down Main Street? The band, the firemen, Girl and Boy Scouts, neighbors and their children riding in their antique cars. It's the kind of town where you hear more than you need to know, hopefully taking it all in with a grain of salt.

Having grown up in the greater New York City metropolitan area, I moved to the northern Catskill Mountains in New York State 25 years ago. It is the place I have chosen to call my true home. I married a "local" and raised my daughter here. She is considered a native because she was born here, but through no fault of my own, I never will be. I am a board certified, state licensed art therapist with an MA in Counseling. I have cobbled together a patchwork of part-time jobs so that I can practice what I love while making an adequate living for my family. I was forced to do this because the insurance reimbursement laws through Medicaid and others will not reimburse some mental health professionals for services, even in this underserved area that has a severe shortage of mental health professionals.

My town is in Delaware County, a county larger than the state of Rhode Island, with a population of about 48,000 and slowly shrinking. It is the second poorest county in New York State, and by most definitions, is very rural.

My town is a typical slice of rural America, the same rural America that accounts for more than 25% of our population and 90% of its land mass. It's the same rural America that supplies the bulk of our food, and which we depend on for most of our water, wool, cotton, lumber, mineral resources, and recreational opportunities. And it houses many descendants of the same rural Americans who built this country in the first place, tree by majestic tree and stone by laden stone. Around here folks like to say there are "two stones for every dirt." Previous generations were known to say that when life gives you rocks, you build rock walls. And when life gives you more rocks, you build those walls higher.

This bucolic countryside is legendary for its beauty, its recreational opportunities, and for the sparkling water that trickles down its mountainsides into the New York City water supply, and that water is 25 square miles in area. A state highway runs through it, slicing one rural village and then another in half. It's not what most people think of as a highway, and is the only two-lane street in town. There are no traffic lights within a dozen miles, nor is there enough traffic to fill a parking lot on the average day. Many roads remain dirt; the dirt is laden with rocks. Although the rocks make farming difficult, the land lends itself to agricultural venues, particularly dairy farming. Thirty years ago, dairy farms were everywhere in this area; now only a handful remain. This was the purple mountain majesty and the fruited plain. Now we have to find another base for our economy.

The gray ribbon of road used to be filled with milk trucks picking up raw milk from farms and delivering it to the local creamery. The creamery remains, but threatens to close at regular intervals.

Roxbury is on the way to nowhere; one must seek it out. Every other town in the area is on the way to somewhere else. Buses run from New York City, 3 hours away, through those towns and on to the college and touristy towns, making them a major thoroughfare, in their two-lane, small town kind of way. Most urbanites have a skewed idea of what rural looks like because they stick to interstate routes.

Too small to be called anything but a hamlet, the center of town has a gas station, a convenience store, a general store, a restaurant, and many empty storefronts. Its people are rugged and determined survivalists. They have to be. The hamlet and surrounding town sit an hour or more away from a movie theater, a chain restaurant, a large hospital, an airport, or department stores. If you need any of these services, you need to hope for good weather or it will be an all-day affair, and perhaps a dangerous one at that. Nevertheless, life goes on in Roxbury, and we often have to make do. Most of us are good at that. Our independent spirits are suited to the rougher edges of rural life.

There is no one-size-fits-all approach that works in rural areas. Rural areas are themselves culturally diverse, often housing pockets of ethnic groups and indigenous populations, making each community unique. Central among the barriers to rural residents getting the treatment they need are accessibility, availability, affordability, and acceptability of services. In addition, our hospitals are either closing or downsizing to become Critical Access Hospitals that provide limited services. Anyone needing to go to an emergency room for a mental health crisis may be out of luck as to whether or not they can be helped appropriately.

Like any other small rural town, life in Roxbury has its challenges. It is at the eastern end of Delaware County, the second poorest county in New York State, with the highest suicide rate in the state. It has a high rate of drug and alcohol abuse, domestic violence, sexual abuse, depression, anxiety, and all the other mental health issues any other town has. Here in these mountains, however, finding services is an uphill climb.

The nearest crisis center is over an hour away. The nearest public mental health facility is an hour away in good weather. The handful of mental health practitioners in the area are in private practice, and the state doesn't allow all of them to take your insurance even though they are licensed and need the work.

The community mental health movement that began in the late 1960s and peaked in the late 1970s affected rural America. For the first time the rural population grew faster than the urban population. We called it the "back to the land movement," propelling the hippie movement to its next logical step. Modern technology has allowed many people's work to be done virtually so they can live wherever they wish. Overnight delivery services can ship whatever cannot be sent virtually via computer, and they even deliver to most dirt roads in my area.

In these early years of the 21st century, the farm crisis that began in the 1980s continues. The number of family-owned farms in the United States has decreased, while the large corporate agribusiness farms supply an ever greater percentage of our food, often with genetically modified seed, insecticides, and cheap labor. How will America care for the quarter of its population it depends on for so much?

1 What Defines Rural and Frontier, and Why Are They Important?

Rural and frontier represents well over 90% of America's land mass and 25% of its population. We rely on rural areas for much in the way of food and natural resources. This chapter explores the myriad formal and informal definitions of rural and frontier and the reasons they are important. It uses Delaware County, New York, as an example of a rural area with no close proximity to a city. The terms behavioral health and mental health are explored and contrasted, and a picture of what exactly a rural mental health practitioner is begins to emerge. The terms urban and rural are explored, as are the terms urbanormativity and urbancentric. The stereotype of rural as a homogeneous group is shattered, and we begin to see a picture of what rural truly consists of.

Formal and Informal Definitions

Rural America is made up of 2,305 counties, contains 90% of our land mass, and is home to over 25% of our population, which is well over 62 million people. Of those rural residents, 17% are minorities. Carr and Kefalas write that without this country's rural residents, the country couldn't function in the same way that a body cannot function without a heart, and that by the end of the 20th century, independent farmers became more like modern-day sharecroppers.

Rural populations are treated as an ethnically and racially homogeneous group when in fact they differ significantly from one area of the country to another, and for that matter, they often differ from town to town. Rurality is its own culture that is unique, differs geographically in different parts of our country, and needs to be treated as a separate culture in consideration of multiculturalism. Sometimes those differences are broader than the diversity between rural and urban populations. So many factors enter into shaping a rural subculture. Climate, daily weather, altitude, natural resources, and agricultural heritage are just a few. Accidents and gun-related crimes are disproportionately higher in rural areas. Chronic diseases and infant mortality rates are also much higher in rural areas. How, then, do we provide the mental health resources this population sorely needs?

Defining Rural and Frontier

There are almost as many definitions of rural as there are states. Some define rural by the number of miles one needs to travel to reach a supermarket or pharmacy; others define it by the number of residents per square mile. The Department of Health and Human Services reports that there is no consistent definition of rural used across federal agencies or programs. In fact, the definitions of rural are so problematic and varied that the US Office of Rural Health Policy issued an entire publication just on the definitions. During the 20th century, the rural population in America shrank from 60% early in the century to about 24% by the century's end.

From a rural land mass point of view, it makes sense to start with a definition of rural and in turn label all external areas as urban. From a spatial standpoint, this makes sense, because most of the land in the United States is in fact rural. This phenomenon of always putting rural at the back of the line is called urbancentric or urbanormativity. In sociological terms, urbanormativity implies that urban is the norm and rural is therefore, by process of elimination, abnormal or deviant.

The federal Office of Management and Budget (OMB) bases its operational definition of rural on county types, putting the most weight on the degree of social and economic interaction between core and adjacent communities, and tend to use "non-metropolitan" as an identifying term rather than "rural." This urbancentric point of view is our federal government's way of viewing our country. Flora and Flora (2008) point out that researchers and policy makers use statistics from both the US Census Bureau and the OMB, which utilize different methods and take into consideration different variables when defining rural. OMB includes the distinctions of metropolitan, non-metropolitan, and micropolitan. The Economic Research Service of the USDA provides yet another definition of rural that includes urban to rural continuum codes in order to overcome the shortcomings of a simpler classification system.

The lead federal agency for rural health is the Office of Rural Health Policy (ORP) under the umbrella of the Department of Health and Human Services (HHS). Every state has a rural affairs office in its capital. In general, the government considers the county as the smallest breakdown of land. However, counties can be a mixture of urban and rural, skewing the statistics and causing confusion. A truer definition would be to consider each community the smallest unit of population measurement. To muddy the water even further, the US Census Bureau considers an urbanized area as having 50,000 people or more with a population density of more than 1,000 per square mile, an urban cluster as having between 2,500 and 50,000 people, and a micropolitan area as having between 10,000 and 50,000 people; rural is everything left over. Ninety-seven percent of our land mass is what is left over.

The Economic Research Service of the USDA uses a much more complex definition of rural that includes rural codes. Using rural upstate New York as an example, towns in New York State are classified as either towns "of the first class," which includes towns with populations over 10,000, or those with over 5,000 who request that status. Towns with over 25,000 people and are within a reasonable proximity to a city are classified as towns "of the second class." However these definitions do not take into account population density. Because of that, counties with larger geographic areas may not be labeled as rural, even if they have fewer residents per square mile than a geographically smaller county with proportionately more residents. Similar disparity arises with nearly every definition of rural.

The vast majority of upstate New York consists of rural and agricultural towns. According to the authors of *Critical Rural Theory*, a typical agricultural town has a landscape marked by the most farm fields, groves of fruit trees, manure ponds, barns, chicken coops, and other agriculturally related buildings. In contrast, a "natural" town has a landscape that has been kept in a more or less natural state.

The generally accepted definition of a frontier is an area with six people or fewer per square mile. Most frontier areas in the United States are subject to regular bouts of severe weather, unfriendly terrain, limited water, or other resources for use by the resident population and for economic growth. I recently visited Alaska and experienced the meaning of the word "vast" firsthand. Even the cities of Fairbanks and Anchorage are tiny by big city standards. While traveling between those two Alaskan cities, I realized that by comparison, Alaska makes my home area look almost urban. Alaska has more caribou than people (and did you know that reindeer are domesticated caribou?), and 40% of its citizens are licensed pilots because of the vastness of their state.

In frontier America, mental health can look different than it does in rural areas. In Alaska, at the level of local village governance, most services are provided by village health aides who work on the paraprofessional level as alcohol and mental health counselors. Although there is a certification system, an extensive training manual and a Village Drug Reference, which is like the PDR (Physicians' Desk Reference) but with a much more simplified list of drugs that can be administered locally with telephone backup from the regional family physician. In remote frontier areas, multiple public agencies are often involved, with overlapping jurisdictions and responsibilities. The result is often confusion and duplication of certain kinds of services and a scarcity of others. If a suicidal person needs to be flown to a hospital, they had better hope the weather is cooperative for flying. And the cost can be prohibitive.

There are two opposing models of rural versus urban points of view. On the one hand is the popular belief that innovations originate in urban areas and spread their way to rural areas. This is what sociologists refer to as the urban-centric point of view. The opposite view is that innovation begins with rural areas contributing the natural resources or raw materials for cultural innovation that are then polished by urban centers. Neither view credits rural areas with innovation. According to Thomas, rural areas are pitched as receiving urban innovations. Rural people are cast as empty vessels passively anticipating new ideas and information. When it comes to mental health, the rate of problems does not differ much between rural and urban areas. It is the experience of these issues that differs drastically.

According to the 2000 census, one in five Americans can be considered rural (www.census.gov/geo/tiger/glossry2.html). Fewer than one-fifth of rural counties in the United States are dependent on agriculture for their economies. And here's a fascinating milestone of humanity: for the first time in human history we've reached the tipping point in which there are more people on our planet living in urban than rural areas. That is an astounding turn of events.

Rural topography in the United States varies from rugged mountainous terrain with snowcapped mountains in summer, to dry, parched deserts, from flat, windy wheat fields to humid wetlands and everything in between. Weather is the wild card in all these areas, especially with climate change creating unprecedented storms and their accompanying floods and droughts. Notice the rampant tornadic activity in the middle and southern parts of the country (although they are not limited to those areas), and the record-setting hurricanes, snowstorms, and rainfall totals of recent years. And although severe weather can happen anywhere, weather outplays almost everything else about rural living, where resources are scant for rebuilding.

Rural Matters: YOU ARE HERE
From a flyer used at a community event.

DELAWARE COUNTY, NEW YORK

Did you know that:

- Delaware County is as large as the state of Rhode Island, measuring in at 1,468 square miles (1,443 land, 25 water) and a population of only 48,000 and steadily shrinking.
- It is equal in area to Los Angeles County, and the distance from one end of the county to another is over 80 miles. There is no public transportation.
- More than two-thirds of the land in Delaware County is owned by New York City and State, most for the purpose of the New York City watershed.
- Delaware County has the lowest population density in New York State outside of the Adirondacks and is home to 48,000 people and dwindling.
- Delaware County is home to 33.2 people per square mile, as compared to a state average of 402 per square mile.
- Delaware County experiences population loss at a rate double to that of the rest of New York State.
- There is presently only one psychiatrist in the county, whose caseload can reach 1,500.

- Nine percent of families and 12.9% of the population lives below the poverty line.
- **Delaware County is the second poorest county in the state.**
- **Delaware County has the highest suicide rate in the state.**

A Few Words on the Terms Behavioral Health and Mental Health

Although the terms behavioral health and mental health are often used interchangeably, they are actually two distinct things. The term behavioral health began to address a combination of mental health and substance abuse. Behavioral health is a blanket term often used to describe the connection between our behaviors and the health and well-being of the body, mind, and spirit. This includes behaviors such as eating, drinking, or exercising that impact physical or mental health either immediately or over a longer period of time. It may also include broader factors such as having to live in an area with high pollution or experiencing high levels of stress over a long period of time. In short, behavioral health looks at how behaviors impact someone's physical and mental health.

Frequently, physical health and mental health issues play off each other and can occur simultaneously. For example, people with cancer or cardiac conditions often develop depression as well. Ultimately, the goals of behavioral health interventions are similar to those of other mental health treatment: helping people function and learn about themselves and their feelings so they can lead healthier, fuller lives.

Mental health is psychological well-being or an absence of mental illness. It is the psychological state of someone who functions at adequate level of emotional adjustment in their actions and relationships. From the perspective of positive psychology, mental health includes a person's ability to enjoy life, create a balance in their life activities, and have an ample supply of psychological resilience and other tools with which to weather emotional storms of various kinds.

What Does a Rural Mental Health Professional Look Like?

Many are the occupational hazards of the rural mental health practitioner. Coping with the rural environment is not to be underestimated. Mother Nature rules the roost, and winters can be long and harsh. All it takes is a dusting of snow to make the roads slippery, and the weather can and does turn on a dime. The locals will tell you if you don't like the weather here, wait 10 minutes. I've seen it happen enough times to know that it is true. Summers are usually beautiful, but not without severe thunderstorms, hailstorms, sizzling hot weeks with full humidity, and even frost in July (rumor has it there was once one in August, but I haven't experienced it myself).

When dealing with community and personal interactions, no one in a rural area has personal privacy. And sometimes rural practitioners must develop ways to cope with situations in order to continue to live and practice in the same small town. But ultimately, the well-being of the individual is tightly bound to the well-being of the community.

When it comes to running and managing a rural private practice, I have several clients who live in the area and have no driver's license (whether revoked or never received) and no automobile. Therefore I decided it was necessary to make home visits in order to serve the really local population. I set limits for the home visits in terms of accessibility, not wanting to travel muddy dirt roads or icy back roads in the winter. Most of those who needed for me to make home visits live in one of the villages, making them highly accessible.

It is of the utmost importance to decode and begin to function within the prevailing rural ethic. That includes ethics, politics, attitudes about diversity, religion, professionals and educational status, socioeconomic status, and lifestyle choices. It also includes some lesser topics such as educational attitudes, sports abilities and interests, the willingness to volunteer for various things, the ability to get to know everyone's automobile and waving whenever we pass them on the road. Also important is the degree of self-reliance you use to run your life. Already struggling with limited resources by definition, rural populations have all they can do to gather the resources necessary to help their own. To make a generalization, it has been my experience that the rural population admires those who keep worries to themselves and take care of their own lives. Gossip is the kiss of death in rural social life. While gossiping might initially make you some friends, very soon no one will trust you because of it. In rural areas, comfort within the therapist/client relationship is determined foremost by the level of trust in the confidentiality factor. While mental health practitioners are trained to think in terms of ambiguity, rural folks have little tolerance for it, wanting straightforward answers. And while mental health professionals by definition believe in the possibility and desirability of change, rural populations often doubt that changes can be made.

Read more about rural mental health professionals in Chapters 9, 11, and 15.

References

Bird, D.C., Dempsey, P., & Hartley, D. (2001). *Addressing mental health workforce needs in underserved rural areas: Accomplishments and challenges.* Portland, ME: Maine Rural Health Research Center.

Brown, D.L., & Schafft, K. (2011). *Rural People and Communities.* Malden, MA: Polity Press.

Brown, D.L., & Swanson, L. (Eds.). (2003). *Challenges for Rural America in the Twenty-First Century.* University Park: Pennsylvania State University Press.

Buettgens, M., & Dev, J. (June, 2014). *Robert Wood Johnson Foundation/Urban Institute.* www.rwjf.org/en/library.

Butler, C., Butler, J., & Gasteyer, S. (2016). *Rural Communities: Legacy and Change* (5th ed.). Boulder, CO: Westview Press.

Carr, P.J., & Kefalas, M.J. (2009). *Hollowing Out the Middle: The Rural Brain Drain and What It Means for America.* Boston: Beacon Press.

Carter, R. (2010). *Within Our Reach: Ending the Mental Health Crisis*. Emmaus, PA: Rodale Books.
Castle, E. (Ed.). (1995). *The Changing American Countryside: Rural People and Places*. Lawrence: University Press of Kansas.
Census.gov/geo/tiger/glossry2.html.
Cloke, P., Marsden, T., & Mooney, P. H. (Eds.). (2006). *Handbook of Rural Studies*. Thousand Oaks, CA: Sage.
Cornell University. (2010). *Poverty, Local and Regional Government, Energy, Economic and Workforce Development, Agriculture and Food Systems*. Ithaca, NY. www.cornell.edu.
Davidson, O. G. (1996). *Broken Heartland: The Rise of America's Rural Ghetto*. Iowa City: University of Iowa Press.
Duncan, C. (1999). *Worlds Apart: Why Poverty Persists in Rural America*. New Haven, CT: Yale University Press.
Elder, G., & Conger, R. (Eds.). (2000). *Children of the Land: Adversity and Success in Rural America*. Chicago: University of Chicago Press.
Fitchen, J. (1991). *Endangered Spaces, Enduring Places*. Boulder, CO: Westview Press.
Flora, C. B., & Flora, J. L. (2008). *Rural Communities, Legacy and Change* (3rd ed.). Philadelphia, PA: Westview Press/Perseus Books.
Lightburn, A., & Sessions, P. (2006). *Handbook of Community-Based Clinical Practice*. New York: Oxford University Press.
Mental Health America. (August 29, 2016). Statement by Paul Gionfriddo, President and CEO, Mental Health America. mhapostmaster@mentalhealthamerica.net.
Mental Health and Rural America: 1994–2005. (2005). Washington, DC: Health Resources and Services Administration, Office of Rural Health Policy.
Mohatt, D. F. (2016). *Rural Mental Health: Challenges and Opportunities Caring For the Country*. Boulder, CO: Western Interstate Commission for Higher Education.
Morris, J. A. (1997). *Practicing Psychology in Rural Settings*. Washington, DC: American Psychological Association.
New Freedom Commission on Mental Health. (2003). *Achieving the Promise: Transforming Mental Healthcare in America*. Final. DHHS Pub. Co. SMA-03–3832. Rockville, MD.
Perry, M. (2002). *Population: 485, Meeting Your Neighbors One Siren at a Time*. New York: Harper Perennial.
Rhodes, P. (Ed.). (2014). *Mental Health and Rural America*. New York: Nova Science.
Sawyer, D., Gale, J., & Lambert, D. (2006). *Rural and Frontier Mental and Behavioral Health Care: Barriers, Effective Policy Strategies, and Best Practices*. Washington, DC: National Association for Rural Mental Health.
Smalley, K. B., Yancey, C. T., Warren, J. C., Naufel, K., Ryan, R., & Pugh, J. L. (2010). Rural mental health and psychological treatment: A review for practitioners. *Journal of Clinical Psychology: In Session*, 66(5), 479–489.
Thomas, A., Lowe, B., Fulkerson, G., & Smith, P. (2011). *Critical Rural Theory: Structure, Space and Culture*. New York: Lexington Books.

2 Rural Mental Health Policy and Parity

This chapter explores policy and parity in rural mental health. Beginning with a timeline of significant mental health developments from 1840 through the present, it focuses on modern developments in the field such as the Institutions for Mental Diseases (IMD) exclusion; Jimmy Carter's President's Commission on Mental Health; George H. W. Bush's Decade of the Brain, which culminated in the President's New Freedom Commission on Mental Health; the Mental Health Parity Act of 2008 and its enforcement; and Barack Obama's Affordable Care Act (ACA) with its implications. It concludes with the development of the 21st Century Cures Act and the Medicaid Redesign Program.

History of Rural Mental Health

The prevalence of adults with serious mental illness and children with serious emotional disturbances is generally similar between rural and urban areas. Research shows repeatedly that lower rates of access to rural mental health services relates directly to lower rates of the availability and supply of mental health providers.

In ancient societies such as the Greek, Roman, Indian, and Egyptian cultures, mental illness was viewed as a religious or personal problem. In the 5th century BC, Hippocrates was a pioneer in treating mentally ill people with techniques not rooted in religion or superstition. Instead, he chose to focus on altering the patient's environment or occupation, or administering what we would consider to be precursors to medication. Moving ahead to the Middle Ages, the mentally ill were believed to be possessed or in need of religion. Negative attitudes toward mental illness were sustained into 18th-century America, which led to keeping the mentally ill locked up, often in asylums, in unsanitary conditions.

A Timeline of Mental Health in Rural America

- 1840s—Dorothea Dix discovered that the mentally ill were kept in dangerous and unhealthy conditions, shut away in institutions.

For the next 40 years, Dix devoted herself to the plight of the mentally ill and eventually persuaded the US government to fund the construction of 32 state psychiatric hospitals throughout the country. At the time, this was considered the most effective way to care for the mentally ill and intellectually disabled. The idea was that by living in an institution, patients had greater access to services, but the reality proved otherwise.

- 1908–1910—Author Clifford Beers's autobiography, *A Mind That Found Itself*, changed society's view on living with serious mental illness. He founded the group that eventually became Mental Health America, which continues to be at the forefront of informing and educating the public on mental health issues.
- 1930—The first International Congress on Mental Hygiene convened. Their goal was educating the public to understand that mental illness is an actual disease. During Franklin Roosevelt's administration, a number of programs were developed to increase chronically low farm incomes, ensure a stable and cheap food supply, and conserve farmland. It was an era that is remembered as the golden age of farm policy or as agriculture's dark years, depending on one's political bias.
- 1946—President Harry Truman passed the National Mental Health Act, which created the National Institute of Mental Health (NIMH), and for the first time in US history, federal funds were earmarked toward research into the causes and treatments for mental illness. It also provided aid to states for developing programs to address mental illness and reduce the need for institutional care, and developed and promoted training for mental health professionals.
- 1950s—A push for deinstitutionalization and the beginning of outpatient treatment and community-oriented care, facilitated in part by the development of a variety of antipsychotic drugs. From this point on, only those who posed a threat to themselves or others would be committed to psychiatric units. The number of institutionalized mentally ill patients fell from its peak of 560,000 in the 1950s to 130,000 by 1980. By the year 2000, the number of psychiatric beds per 100,000 people was 22, down from 339 in 1955.
- 1952—Thorazine, the first antipsychotic medicine for mental illnesses such as schizophrenia, became available on the market. Tricyclic antidepressants and monoamine oxidase inhibitors for depression became available to consumers.
- 1955—Congress votes to enact the National Mental Health Act to establish and expand existing programs.

- Early 1960s Benzodiazepines to treat anxiety enter the marketplace.
- 1963—President Kennedy became the first world leader to publicly discuss mental illness and mental retardation. He signed into law the Maternal and Child Health and Mental Retardation Planning Amendment, which focused on prevention, as well as the bill for the Construction of Mental Retardation Facilities and Community Mental Health Centers. These provided federal funding for the development of community-based mental health services and the establishment of county mental health clinics. This legislation in effect mandated deinstitutionalization for all except those who posed an imminent danger to themselves or others, and provided an alternative. The overall aim of this legislation was to substitute comprehensive community care for institutional care in order to save money. Kennedy believed that poverty was a primary causal factor in mental illness, and this new program would create community prevention programs specifically aimed at low-income people. He also proposed a 50% reduction in state hospital populations across the country over the next 10 years.
- 1965—Medicare and Medicaid were born. They contained an exclusionary clause called Institutions for Mental Diseases (IMD), which was designed to help hasten the emptying of mental illness hospitals so they could be closed, according to Patrick Kennedy. Both Medicaid and Medicare contained provisions for mental health care, but stays in state hospitals were not covered and mentally ill people under the age of 65 were ineligible for Medicaid benefits. These provisions resulted in the transfer of large numbers of the elderly who were mentally ill from state hospitals to nursing homes.
- 1965—President Lyndon Johnson's Social Security Amendments of 1965 included the creation of the Joint Commission on the Mental Health of Children.
- Late 1960s to 1970s—The issues associated with the policy of discharging mass numbers of people from state hospitals, or deinstitutionalization were being realized and were numerous and serious. There simply were not enough community facilities to handle those numbers of people, and far from enough well-trained staff. The terminology for referring to residents were moron, idiot, or imbicile. Many were deliberately exposed to Hepatitis B. Investigative reporters built careers on discovering filthy, poorly run institutions, such as those in the Willowbrook facility in Staten Island, New York (a state institution for the mentally ill or developmentally delayed children). Robert Kennedy had called it a "snake pit" in 1965, and Geraldo Rivera released his famous expose of the facility in 1972. It wasn't officially closed until 1987.

- 1977—President Jimmy Carter passed the Commission on Mental Health, raised the importance of the mental health status of the nation's citizens, and sought recommendations on ways to improve mental health treatment. The president's wife, Rosalynn, chose mental health as the issue she would champion and started the Carter Foundation for the purpose of mental health research, dissemination of information, and assistance with mental health policy issues.
- 1979—The National Alliance for the Mentally Ill (NAMI) was founded to provide support, education, research, and advocacy for those with serious psychiatric illnesses. It remains a strong force in advocating for the mentally ill.
- Ronald Reagan won the 1980 presidential election with promises to reduce government waste and regulation while returning the responsibility for many social programs to the states.
- 1981—Known as the new federalism, President Reagan passed the Omnibus Budget Reconciliation Act (OBRA) of 1981, which repealed the Mental Health Systems Act, shrinking the role of the federal government in mental health affairs to that of mere technical assistance, passing the responsibility down to the states and local communities.
- 1987—The first selective serotonin reuptake inhibitors (SSRIs) Prozac, Paxil, and Zoloft became available to treat depression and anxiety.
- 1990—The Americans with Disabilities Act was passed to prohibit, once and for all, discrimination in any form against those with physical and mental disabilities.
- 1996—Mental Health Parity Act—passed in order to require insurance companies to provide equal coverage for mental health issues as they would for any physical illness.
- 2002—President George W. Bush created the President's New Freedom Commission on Mental Health, which focused on investigating the problems and finding solutions to themes such as ending stigma, fixing the fragmented mental health care system, and addressing unfair disparities in mental health insurance coverage. The Commission found that the vast majority of Americans living in rural and remote areas were underserved, and as a result experienced disparities in mental health services compared to those living in urban areas. The Commission concluded that rural issues are often minimized, misunderstood, and ignored in discussions leading to the formulation of mental health policy. At President Bush's last State of the Union address, he did not mention mental illness at all, and followed it up with a proposed budget cut of $88 million in funding for mental health programs.

- 2008—The Wellstone Domenici Mental Health Parity and Addiction Equity Act expanded federal requirements for mental health insurance coverage. Insurance companies now needed to cover mental illness in equal measure with physical health for those who work for businesses with more than 50 employees. Unfortunately this is a minority of rural residents.
- 2010—The Patient Protection and Affordable Care Act of 2010 passed. This landmark legislation, more commonly known as the Affordable Care Act (ACA), mandates insurance for all citizens. It also eliminates a lifetime cap for a person's medical expenses and mandates that insurance cover pre-existing conditions. It also allows young adults to stay on their parent's plans until age 26. Prior to the ACA, rural families paid up to 50% of their health care costs out of pocket, and this when one in five farmers is in debt. Among the resources the ACA adds to rural areas is more funding for community health centers; it also expands the funding for loan repayment scholarships to encourage more health professionals to practice in rural areas and additional funds for rural hospitals and clinics and telemedicine costs. The ACA is a landmark in social policy, comparable to Roosevelt's New Deal and the creation of Medicare and Medicaid in the 1960s. Although President Obama, himself a Democrat, said he knew the bill had flaws, he was able to get it passed through both houses of Congress in spite of the fact that they were dominated by the Republican party and worked hard to block his legislation.

In June 2013, President Obama hosted the National Conference on Mental Health in order to increase the understanding and awareness of mental health issues in America. Conference attendees included people from a wide range of professions including members of Congress, local government officials, individuals who have battled mental illness themselves, faith leaders, educators, mental health professionals of all kinds, and health care providers. Reducing stigma was at the top of the agenda as well as increasing mental health services for veterans. The administration continued to implement the Affordable Care Act (ACA), which builds on the Mental Health Parity and Addiction Equity Act of 2008 and expanded mental health and substance use disorder benefits and federal parity protections for 62 million Americans.

The federal government was already paying attention to mental illness, having passed a law in 1955—cosponsored by a young senator by the name of John F. Kennedy—establishing the Joint Commission on Mental Illness and Mental Health. In early 1963, JFK delivered his landmark "Special Message to the Congress on Mental Illness and Mental Retardation." It represented the first time that either of these medical conditions ever had been discussed in public by a world that preferred to pretend that they existed. Kennedy, whose sister Rosemary was what was then referred to as mentally retarded, knew firsthand of the trials and tribulations of that kind of disability. He called for "a new approach to mental illness and mental retardation," and said that the coldness of institutional care would be supplanted by the open warmth of community concern and capability. On October 31, he signed what was now called the bill for the Construction of Mental Retardation Facilities and Community Mental Health Centers. Three weeks after that landmark legislation was signed, JFK was assassinated.

The original 1963 federal legislation that created Community Mental Health Centers stipulated that each center receiving federal funds must employ a psychiatrist, psychologist, social worker, and nurse, and recommended that professionals in other related disciplines involved with the rehabilitation of those with mental illness also be involved. There was clear recognition of the value of professional perspectives, and the centers were mandated to develop and maintain strong ties to the communities they served. The centers created governing boards representative of various community agencies and stakeholders. Advisory boards also provided input and helped create collaborative relationships with a broader range of professionals and others interested in mental health.

In some locations, these agencies exist as self-supporting and relatively comprehensive mental health centers; in others they may be agencies contracted to state or county government to provide mental health services. And in others, the mental health provider may be an employee of the county's human services program. That model holds true today, and is called a Community Services Board (CSB). Although these advances were revolutionary in their time, half a century later there are still obstacles to collaboration and teamwork within the mental health system.

Barriers to collaboration can be structural or personal. Structural barriers consist of characteristics of institutions or systems of care that impede collaborative work between persons of different disciplines. Personal barriers consist of characteristics of the person or groups of professional persons that prevent collaborative work.

In the early 1960s, the farm poor were without a real voice. Most middle-class Americans viewed the government giving aid to farmers as a vast waste of money, a Robin Hood technique for robbing millions of urbanites and giving to the poor countryside. Yet poor farmers did not receive a cent; they were simply left out.

Simultaneously, mental health professionals were starting to rethink the diagnosis, treatment, and underlying causes of mental illness. The results came in the form of a landmark revision of the DSM, the *Diagnostic and Statistical Manual of Mental Disorders*, considered the bible for psychiatric diagnosis in the United States. Published by the American Psychiatric Association, the DSM was originally published in the 1950s as an expanded version of the mental health section of the World Health Organization's standardized listing of every known illness.

By the time the DSM-III came into being, it had gone from being an obscure technical manual to a bestselling book used by teachers, doctors, lawyers, and judges to make sense of the dynamic, expanding field of psychiatric diagnosis. Now when a diagnosis was made, there was a clear standard set. It remained a medical model and continued to be highly supported by the pharmaceutical industry. Although it helped clarify the symptomology into diagnosis, the lines between diagnosis and non-diagnosis were drawn arbitrarily to, say, three of five of the symptoms listed.

Patrick Kennedy, former congressman from Rhode Island and son of Senator Ted Kennedy, writes in *A Common Struggle* that the Institutions for Mental Diseases (IMD) exclusion is a law from the 1960s meant to prevent dilapidated facilities from refilling their beds when Medicare/Medicaid was passed. This antiquated law prevents many facilities from getting Medicaid reimbursement for patients between the ages of 22 and 64. The original purpose of the IMD exclusion was to prevent the "snake pits" that housed people with mental illness from perpetuating mistreatment with federal funding. Kennedy firmly believes that the IMD exclusion is a gross parity violation with no valid justification for its continued existence. Congress must also eliminate Medicare's arbitrary 190-day lifetime limit on inpatient psychiatric hospital care—a restriction that does not exist for any other inpatient Medicare service. This limit is particularly harmful for adults between the ages of 22 and 64 who are eligible for both Medicaid and Medicare because of disability status. Many of these individuals with psychiatric conditions are gravely disabled and will likely need more than 190 days of inpatient care throughout their lifetimes. This era in mental health is significant because the situation became so awful that consumers, out of sheer frustration, created the modern consumer medical advocacy movement as it is known now. The silver lining was that those years in mental health were so bad they encouraged the consumer advocacy we take for granted in the field today.

When Jimmy Carter took office in 1977, one of his first acts in office was to create the President's Commission on Mental Health. Rosalynn Carter was named the honorary chair of the commission. Mental health is a cause she championed and continues to devote herself to through the organization she founded called the Carter Center. She wanted those with mental health issues to receive the same funding and protections as those with developmental disabilities. Her main focus was on those suffering from serious mental illnesses and who are not responding to treatments or are unable to stay on them and therefore often end up disabled, homeless, or in prison. Her goal was to publicize the cause and the need, which she hoped would lead to a broad bill that would help everyone suffering from a brain disorder.

The commission's hearings addressed many of the problems identified in JFK's Community Mental Health Act that had remained unsolved—or in some cases had actually worsened—since that historic legislation. Deliberations went on for more than a year and drew an incredibly broad cast of characters, most of whom agreed on almost nothing. This was partly because, in an attempt to be broadly "inclusive" at a time before a true medical understanding of mental illnesses had emerged, every social, ethnic, and gender issue that might produce psychological stressors was included in their discussions.

One of the most significant advancements in mental health was the establishment of the federal Office of Rural Health Policy and the National Rural Health Advisory Committee in 1987 within the Health Resources and Services Administration.

In 1989, George H.W. Bush declared the "Decade of the Brain." His idea was to force teamwork between the federal agencies, powerful institutions, clinicians in the field, and companies that focus on neurological and psychiatric illness and "admit they are all dealing with the same brain." Unfortunately, President Bush and Congress neglected to attach any increase in funding to it. According to Patrick Kennedy, the Decade of the Brain wasn't even an underfunded mandate—it was really no mandate at all. Bush deliberately placed the medicine and science of mental health and addiction back under the oversight of the National Institutes of Health (NIH) in the hopes that it would be taken more seriously and attract larger amounts of funding. This had a huge ripple effect in the way both the government and the general public viewed mental illness.

At the same time, Prozac burst onto the scene. This created a huge buzz of excitement throughout the country as it was touted as highly effective with few side effects. Shortly after Prozac was available on the open market, other SSRIs began to appear, giving significant hope to many suffering with chronic depression, anxiety, and other mental illnesses. In addition, Clozaril arrived on the market as the first atypical antipsychotic medication for treating schizophrenia and schizoaffective disorders—a huge leap forward in the treatment of psychotic disorders.

In 2002, President George W. Bush created the President's New Freedom Commission on Mental Health. He charged the commission, made up of 22 members, with making a comprehensive study of the mental health service delivery system and make recommendations that would enable adults with serious mental illnesses and children with serious emotional disturbance to live, work, learn, and participate fully in their communities. The commission, after a year of reviewing research and testimony, found that the promise of the New Freedom Initiative—a life in the community for everyone—can be realized. Yet for too many Americans with mental illnesses, the mental health services and supports they need remain fragmented, disconnected, and often inadequate, frustrating the opportunity for recovery. Today's mental health care system is a piecemeal relic—the outcome of fragmented policies. Instead of ready access to quality care, the system presents barriers that all too often add to the burden of mental illnesses for individuals, their families, and our communities. It was unclear how Bush planned to solve the Republican roadblock of cost.

The commission also concluded that the best approach to mental health reform needs to be the antithesis of the prior piecemeal approaches. They recommended a fundamental transformation of the nation's approach to mental health care, one that must ensure that mental health services and supports actively facilitate recovery, and build resilience in people in order to face life's challenges. Too often, the system simply managed symptoms and accepted long-term disability for people rather than real recovery. This will require genuine collaborative efforts from all stakeholders involved with the mental health system. The commission came up with an 8-point listing of suggestions for high-quality mental health care at the interface of general medicine and mental health. They include:

- Educated, prepared consumers, primary care providers, and mental health providers.
- Efficient and effective methods to identify, diagnose, and monitor common mental health care at the interface between general medicine and mental health.
- Performance criteria for quality of mental health care at the interface between general medicine and mental health.
- Evidence-based treatment protocols that match treatment intensity to clinical outcomes.
- Trained mental health providers who can support primary care providers with education, proactive follow-up, care management, psychotherapy, and consultation for patients who do not respond to first-line treatments in primary care.
- Effective mechanisms to refer patients who do not improve with treatment in primary care to specialty mental health care and to coordinate care between primary care and specialty mental health care.
- Financing mechanisms for evidence-based models of care for common mental disorders in primary care, including payment for care management, consultation, and supervision of mental health care managers by qualified mental health specialists; psychotherapy at co-payment rates equal to those for the treatment of physical disorders; and prescription medications for mental disorders.

The commission also came up with policy recommendations for overcoming barriers and facilitating use of evidence-based quality improvement models. They include the following points:

- Financing of collaborative care services:
  - Medicare, Medicaid, the Department of Veterans Affairs, other federal- and state-sponsored health insurance programs as well as private insurers should pay for evidence-based collaborative care at the interface of general medicine and mental health, including funding of case management for common mental disorders, supervision of case managers, and consultations to primary care providers by qualified mental health specialists that do not have to involve face-to-face contact with patients.
  - The government should achieve better coordination of the funding and the clinical care provided to clients of publicly funded community clinics for medical, mental, and substance use disorders.

- The federal government should study financial incentives to improve quality of care particularly in the area of mental health care at the interface of mental health and general medicine.
- Performance standards:
    - Federal and state government agencies, private insurers, and accrediting organizations, such as the National Committee for Quality Assurance and the Joint Commission on Accreditation of Healthcare Organizations, should develop clear performance standards for the care of individuals with mental health disorders at the interface of general medicine and mental health. These standards should include appropriate process and outcome indicators.
    - Performance standards should also be developed for the recognition and care of common medical disorders among individuals with severe mental illness, who are often treated primarily in the specialty mental health care sector.
- Technical assistance:
    - Government agencies, such as the Agency for Healthcare Research and Quality, the National Institute of Mental Health, the Substance Abuse and Mental Health Services Administration, the Health Resources and Service Administration, the Department of Veterans Affairs, large insurers, and provider organizations, should develop technical assistance programs to help health care providers implement and disseminate evidence-based models to improve care at the interface of general medicine and mental health.
    - A national technical assistance center should be created to support quality improvement activities at the interface of general medicine and mental health.
- Provider training:
    - National leadership is needed to help improve the training of medical and mental health practitioners in the care of patients at the interface of general medicine and mental health (Transforming MH Services, p. 6).

Historically, rural America lacked the necessary political influence to promote effective rural mental health policy agendas. Senator Byron Dorgan, who served in Congress from 1986 to 2011, is from rural North Dakota. In 2003, he and nine other senators introduced a bill called the New Homestead Act, which specifically targeted communities with declining populations. The sponsors of the bill wanted to rekindle the spirit of the Homestead Act of 1862 and enact policies that offer hope and opportunity to rural America including incentives to buy a home, pay for college, and get the financing to launch or expand a business. The bill offered individuals repayment of up to $10,000 of college loans for people who live and work in rural America for at least five years, a $5,000 tax credit for people who buy homes in rural

America, and created individual homestead accounts, similar to individual retirement accounts. The bill died in 2003. A revised version died in 2005.

In 2005 the Rural Renaissance Act was introduced to Congress. Had it passed, it would have allocated $50 billion in grants and loans for such things as water holding areas and wastewater plants, protect wildlife habitat, soil erosion, preserve air quality, affordable housing, telecommunications, police and fire facilities, hospitals and nursing homes, and renewable fuels projects, including any project to assist agricultural producers in complying with federal, state, or local regulations. It would have also allocated money for value-added agriculture or renewable energy facility projects for agricultural producers or farmer-owned entities, including any project to promote the production or processing of ethanol, biodiesel, animal waste, biomass, raw commodities, or wind as a fuel, a venture capital project for, among others, farmer-owned entities, distance learning or telemedicine projects, and projects to expand broadband technology, something still absent in many rural areas. This version of the bill was defeated and was defeated again in a watered-down variation in 2006. The Rural Renaissance Act, introduced by Lindsay Graham of South Carolina, intended to issue bonds to finance qualified projects for rebuilding areas and amended the Internal Revenue Code to allow a tax credit for investment in bonds, but it died in a similar way.

President George W. Bush is responsible for creating the President's New Freedom Commission on Mental Health. Once established, the commission set out an 8-point plan of goals. These include:

- To continue to build the science base
- To help overcome stigma regarding mental health
- To improve public awareness of effective treatments
- To ensure the supply of evidence-based services and providers trained in evidence-based practices
- To ensure the delivery of state-of-the-art treatments
- To help tailor treatment to age, sex, race, and culture
- To facilitate entry into these treatments
- To reduce financial barriers to getting treatment.

The Mental Health Parity Act of 2008 and the Difficulties in Enforcing Parity

The Mental Health Parity Act of 2008 extended parity for mental health and substance use disorder benefits to large private insurance plans that cover 50 or more people, and if benefits are offered, parity is mandatory. It was the biggest piece of mental health legislation to come along in decades.

The current state of affairs for mental health is not on par with the rest of health care in many areas, namely timely access to care, care coordinators, disease surveillance, research funding, switching to electronic medical records, ways in which law enforcement and the criminal justice system interface with people with behavioral health subconditions, and investment in early intervention, just to name a few, says the Kennedy Forum's Guide for the 115th

Congress. Encouraging compliance with mental health parity is akin to adding enhanced consumer protection to the field.

One of the nation's most successful legislative efforts has been the drive for parity or equality between physical and mental health where it concerns insurance payments. Parity laws have been enacted by 34 states and the federal government—a landmark achievement, but ironically less money is being spent on mental health today than before there were parity laws. Maybe when mental health becomes established as an integral part of health care and is funded as part of health care, the funding amount will be appropriate. Research into systems where behavioral care providers are co-located with primary care physicians reveals that 85% to 90% of patients identified as needing psychological services will accept that help because they can merely walk the short distance down the hall to the office of the mental health provider.

After a long, difficult fight in Congress, the final version of the parity bill was very watered down. It only included serious mental health illnesses, didn't include substance use disorders at all, and the final version even allowed employers to shift the additional costs to employees by raising their co-payments or deductibles. This original mental health parity act was limited, largely because of fear of skyrocketing costs and lack of political will. The mental health community was deeply divided over it, and the public perception of mental health care as scientific and evidence based was under attack.

In 1999, a draft of the first-ever Surgeon General's report on mental health began quietly gathering comments. This 500-page report was put together by an accomplished cast of characters from all corners of the mental health care system. They devoted hundreds of hours to this project as an attempt to create one large document that would explain the challenging history of treating brain diseases and the current state of treatment in lay language regarding research, facilities, caregivers, and patients. It laid out a conceptual road map for change.

Much to the utter astonishment of Rhode Island Congressman Patrick Kennedy (D-RI), he found himself well into the fifth year since the Mental Health Parity Act had been passed, and there was still no end in sight in the battle to get the government to issue the final rules. Interim rules had been introduced in early 2010, but they were not clearly spelled out. They even created some fear because laws are in the details, and because the committee who worked on the bill had left a number of issues unresolved, he was increasingly worried that consumers could lose because of improper interpretation.

The Affordable Care Act (ACA)

In 2010, the Affordable Care Act (ACA) offered extended parity for mental health and substance use disorder benefits to all qualified health insurance plans operated through state health insurance marketplaces, all Medicaid expansion plans, and all individual plans offered after July 1, 2014. According to a study conducted by the Urban Institute and AARP, the ACA's Medicaid expansion was key to reducing the uninsured rate among those aged 50–64 from nearly 12% to 8% in 2014. Ron Manderscheid of the National Association of County Behavioral Health & Developmental Disability Directors

(NACBHDD) reported that more than 2 million people aged 50–64 gained coverage between December 2013 and December 2014. In states that have not expanded Medicaid, the uninsured rate was twice as high as for those who live in expansion states. According to the Department of Health and Human Services, about 137 million individuals, including 55 million women and 28 million children, now have private health insurance covering recommended preventive services without cost sharing. Under the ACA, most health plans are required to provide coverage for recommended preventive health care services without co-pays. Among the preventive services not available is screening for depression and other behavioral problems.

This landmark legislation stipulates that benefits must be offered to all and parity is mandatory. If fact, the bill has a built in monetary penalty for those who refuse to sign on to a health insurance plan. It also demands that financial requirements such as coinsurance and quantitative treatment limitations, which might limit the number of visits to a mental health provider, imposed on mental health and substance use disorder benefits cannot be more restrictive than the predominant financial requirements and quantitative treatment limitations that apply to substantially all medical/surgical benefits. Manderscheid explains that non-quantitative treatment limitations such as benefit management imposed on mental health and substance use disorder benefits cannot be more restrictive than the non-quantitative treatment limitations that apply to substantially all medical and surgical benefits, except for plans that involve 50 or fewer employees and plans that have 1% or more in increased costs for the upcoming year. Criteria for medical necessity determinations in mental health or substance abuse use disorder benefits must be made available upon request to any current or potential plan participant, beneficiary, or contracting provider. The agencies assessing compliance will be the Department of Health and Human Services (HHS) and the Department of Labor (DOL). Compliance will also need to be monitored by each state.

Implications of the Affordable Care Act

- Over 20 million Americans have gained coverage as a result of the ACA, driving the share of Americans without health insurance to the lowest level in history.
- The share of hospitalizations for substance use or mental health disorders in which the patient was uninsured fell from 22% in the fourth quarter of 2013 (just before the ACA's major coverage provisions took effect) to about 14% by the end of 2014.
- In states that expanded Medicaid under the ACA, the uninsured share of substance use or mental health disorder hospitalizations fell from about 20% in the fourth quarter of 2013 to about 5% by mid-2015.

- Between 2010 and 2015, the share of people foregoing mental health care due to cost has fallen by about one-third for people below 400% of the federal poverty level.
- The states with the highest drug overdose deaths also are projected to experience dramatic increases in their uninsured rates if the ACA were repealed: the top three—West Virginia, New Hampshire, and Kentucky—would see their uninsured rates nearly or more than triple if the ACA were repealed, as would Massachusetts (Office of Assistant Secretary for Planning and Evaluation, US Department of Health and Human Services issue brief, January 11, 2017).
- Medicaid funded 25% of all mental health spending and 21% of all addiction spending by any payer in 2014. Limits on Medicaid coverage could set back efforts to treat individuals with behavioral health concerns (Kaiser flyer, 2017).
- Private health insurance has not kept up with the mental health needs of rural residents. The fact is that people who qualify for Medicaid are often better off in terms of mental health care coverage than rural residents who pay for their own private insurance. Unlike many private insurers, Medicaid covers mental health services whether they are delivered in the home, school, or place of work. There are also some special services for acute cases that provide more services to Medicaid recipients.

The Medicare Telehealth Parity Act of 2014 aims to expand reimbursement regarding qualified technologies and types of providers. The act's introduction states that reimbursement mechanisms for telehealth services have been made a priority. Some policy recommendations include allowing for specialized telemedicine licenses at the state level with the license portability to go along with it in order to practice across state lines and establishing online security and safety policies for virtual visits. Enhancing policies and allocating specific funding for the infrastructure of rural broadband needs to happen first so the rest can follow.

In January 2016, President Obama unveiled a set of executive actions against gun violence. Under the new plan, he appealed to Congress to provide $500 million in funding for mental health treatment, to increase the workforce in the field, and make mental health care more accessible. He also directed the Social Security Administration to make its records available for gun background checks, including information about people who have a documented mental illness and are unable to manage their own government benefits. Those individuals will be prohibited from purchasing guns unless they are successful in appealing the process.

The recently signed 21st Century Cures Act requires the Department of Labor and the Departments of Treasury and Health and Human Services to devise an action plan for enhanced parity implementation. The Centers for Disease Control and Prevention (CDC) will establish a broad behavioral health surveillance system so that we have accurate, regularly updated information and statistics on all aspects of the epidemics of mental illness and substance use disorder, including prevalence rates, types of treatment being used, availability of care, and comorbidities with other illnesses the CDC already covers. The work that the CDC already does on incidence of suicide and some other discrete areas of mental health and addiction, the National Survey on Drug Use and Health done by the Substance Abuse and Mental Health Services Administration (SAMHSA), and other smaller efforts are simply not sufficient for public officials, or the public, to understand and track the personal and societal costs. Parity is about more than insurance; we also need parity in epidemiology.

On the other hand, the National Rifle Association (NRA) has backed one bill that includes a provision relating to firearm background checks for the mentally ill. This bill would clarify language regarding the mental health records that are uploaded to national background check system and address the process to restore the ability to purchase a firearm. There is no new innovation here, just clarification. The saddest part of the whole debate is that as of this writing, nothing has been passed or changed. And as a society, we must be careful not to blame the mentally ill for every gun crime in our country. The two go hand in hand in some cases, but there are many more in which the shooter has no mental health record. And then there is the gun control debate, which is a subject that needs and deserves books of its own.

In addition, pitifully few training programs in the mental health field include anything about mental health policy or parity, or for that matter rural culture, making those who do choose to practice in rural areas ill-prepared.

The Cures Act of 2016

The 21st Century Cures Act was signed into law in December 2016 by outgoing President Barack Obama. This bipartisan bill, a rarity in the stalled Congress of its day, weighed in at almost a thousand pages. The Senate passed the 21st Century Cures Act with a 94–5 vote. With just days left in President Obama's term, the House of Representatives passed the bill 392–26 at a time when many thought bipartisanship was dead. Also known as H.R. 34, this act includes provisions from several previous mental health bills that failed; it raises the stature of mental health and substance abuse disorder services at the federal level by creating a new position, Assistant Secretary for Mental Health and Substance Use. It authorized grants for law enforcement and other first responders for de-escalation training, clarifies that Medicaid permits same-day billing for the provision of mental health and primary care services, and required new federal guidance on compliance with mental health and substance use disorder parity requirements.

The first section of this act makes changes to the leadership and oversight by SAMHSA by creating an Assistant Secretary for Mental Health and Substance

Use (ASMHSU), to be appointed by the president and approved by Senate vote. The idea is to enhance collaboration with other agencies, such as the Veterans Administration, the attorney general and the Secretary of Defense.

The other sections of the act include new planning and evaluation requirements, and changes in reporting and accounting requirements. It addresses primarily oversight and accountability issues, as well as better dissemination of data on evidence-based programs and practices. While many applaud this legislation and call it landmark, others express concern that the bill could raise the risk of harmful treatments getting to the marketplace. The bill strengthens privacy protections for participants in genetic research, promotes more pediatric research, and improves the use of electronic health records. Many hope it will speed the development and delivery of promising new treatments for patients. While there is more praise than objection, many feel it gives big pharma and other medical product companies too much flexibility and fear they will lower their product standards. Another provision of the bill is appropriating money for the BRAIN Initiative, a project designed to create new technologies that will assist scientists in mapping the brain with more precision and understanding. The initiative's aim is to discover new ways to prevent, treat, and cure brain disorders like traumatic brain injury (TBI), Alzheimer's disease and other forms of dementia, mental illness, autism, and epilepsy. The hope is that this knowledge will in turn shed light on the complex links between brain function and behavior.

Yet another facet of the act is called the Corrections and Mental Health Collaboration Act, which reauthorizes grants and programs that will improve the interface between corrections agencies and mental health services for the millions of people with behavioral health conditions who become incarcerated. This accounts for almost three-quarters of all persons in county and city jails. It will expand initiatives to provide mental health treatment instead of incarceration through mental health courts, drug courts and others. It is also designed to provide a higher level of support for individuals re-entering the community in order to treat people effectively and lower recidivism rates.

According to NAMI, this legislation will help promote a patient-centered mental health care system in America. Now we are one step closer to NAMI's vision of an America where fewer people with mental illness end up on the streets, out of school, or in jail. NAMI made a public statement that "the battle is won, but the fight is not over." It remained to be seen how these mental health services and supports would be implemented by the new administration in 2017.

The Implications of Medicaid Redesign

Behavioral health conditions, which include both mental illness and addictions, affect a substantial portion of the US population, including many people who have their coverage through Medicaid. A growing number of health providers no longer accept any insurance, which is a barrier to accessing services for millions of people. Medicaid coverage facilitates access to a variety of behavioral health services, including psychiatric evaluations, prescription medication, inpatient treatment, case management, and supportive housing. The Medicaid expansion provides each of the 32 states that signed on to the plan with additional resources to cover behavioral health services for many children and adults who were previously excluded from the program. Between 2014 and 2016, the federal government paid for 100% of the cost of the expansion, and in 2020 and beyond, they will pay for 90% of the expansion. The ACA's Medicaid expansion will add just 2.8% to what states spend on Medicaid, while providing health coverage to 17 million more low-income adults and children. In doing so, the Medicaid expansion will produce savings in state and local government costs for uncompensated care, which will offset at least some of the added state Medicaid costs. Federal support will phase down slightly over the following several years, and by 2020, and for all subsequent years, the federal government will pay 90% of the costs of covering these individuals. Between 2014 and 2022, the federal government will pay $931 billion of the cost of the Medicaid expansion, while states will pay roughly $73 billion, or 7%. As of the time of publication of this book, 19 states have not signed on to the expansion program. To determine if your state has implemented Medicaid expansion, go to www.familiesusa.org.

In a report titled *The ACA and America's Cities: Fewer Uninsured and More Medicaid*, some cities could see a 52% reduction in the number of uninsured. The report states that in some cities the ACA was on track to reduce the number of uninsured residents by 49% and as much as 66% by the end of 2016.

Medicaid restructuring, as proposed in the pending legislation from the Trump administration called the American Health Care Act, and other attempts to repeal Obamacare could limit the ability of states to care for people with behavioral conditions and leave millions uninsured. Some with behavioral health conditions qualify for Medicaid because they have a qualifying disability; others gained coverage through the Medicaid expansion.

What Does Rural Mental Health Look Like Now?

Here are some surprising statistics about rural mental health and mental health in general:

1. Fewer than 10% of rural Americans live on farms.
2. Half of those families have income from off-farm activities.
3. Non-farm employment accounts for nearly 80% of rural jobs.
4. Rural employment income is less than in urban areas.
5. Rural working families are likely to be poorer than urban working families.

6. Over 25% of rural workers over age 25 earn less than the federal poverty rate of $18,390.
7. Depression in adults accounts for almost 400 million sick days a year in the U.S. (Carter), while the number of sick days due to anxiety disorders, post-traumatic stress disorder (PTSD), and substance abuse is a staggering 1.3 billion days of work each year.
8. Children of color are at particular risk, with 46.3% of rural African American children, 43% of rural Native American children, and 41.2% of rural Hispanic children living in poverty.
9. Six hundred (23%) of rural counties are classified as persistent poverty counties by the US government.
10. The younger population is leaving its rural communities, resulting in the elderly population constituting a disproportionate percentage of the remaining population.
11. Over half of rural children are in female-headed families living in poverty.
12. Child poverty is higher in rural areas than in urban areas.
13. About one in five adults nationwide over 18 has a diagnosable mental disorder.
14. Mental illnesses are more common than cancer, diabetes, or heart disease (US Surgeon General's Report).
15. Those who are married, more educated, and Caucasian were more willing to seek mental health treatment.
16. Mental illnesses can affect people of any age, income, religion, race, culture, or gender (National Alliance for the Mentally Ill, or NAMI).
17. Mental illnesses often appear for the first time during adolescence and young adulthood. The young and the elderly are especially vulnerable (NAMI).
18. Four of the 10 leading causes of disability in the United States and other developed countries are mental disorders, which include depression, bipolar disorder, schizophrenia, and obsessive-compulsive disorder. Many people have what practitioners refer to as "comorbid" diagnoses (NAMI).
19. With proper care and treatment, between 70% and 90% of people with mental illnesses experience a significant reduction of symptoms and an improved quality of life (NAMI).

References

Alliance for Health Policy (AHP). (2017). *Essentials of Health Policy: A Sourcebook for Journalists and Policymakers.* www.sourcebook.allhealth.org.

Bagalman, E. (2016). *The Helping Families in Mental Health Crisis Reform Act of 2016.* Washington, DC: Congressional Research Service.

Brown, D. L., & Schafft, K. (2011). *Rural People and Communities*. Malden, MA: Polity Press.

Brown, D., & Swanson, L. (Eds.). (2003). *Challenges for Rural America in the Twenty-First Century*. University Park: Pennsylvania State University Press.

Carter, R. (2010). *Within Our Reach: Ending the Mental Health Crisis*. Emmaus, PA: Rodale Books.

Centers for Disease Control and Prevention (CDC). (2011). *Public Health Action Plan to Integrate Mental Health Promotion and Mental Illness Prevention, 2011–2015*. Atlanta, GA: US Department of Health and Human Services.

Coalition for Mental Health Reform (CMHR). (July 6, 2016). *Concerns With the Helping Families in Mental Health's Crisis Act of 2015—Passed in the House of Representatives*.

Cornell University. (2010). *Poverty, Local and Regional Government, Energy, Economic and Workforce Development, Agriculture and Food Systems*. Ithaca, NY. www.cornell.edu.

Davidson, O. G. (1996). *Broken Heartland: The Rise of America's Rural Ghetto*. Iowa City: University of Iowa Press.

Fitchen, J. (1991). *Endangered Spaces, Enduring Places*. Boulder, CO: Westview Press.

Flora, C. B., & Flora, J. L. (2008). *Rural Communities, Legacy and Change* (3rd ed.). Philadelphia, PA: Westview Press/Perseus Books.

Goldman, H. H., Buck, J. A., & Thompson, K. S. (2009). *Transforming Mental Health Services: Implementing the Federal Agenda for Change*. Arlington, VA: American Psychiatric Association.

Grantham, D. (February 1, 2017). National Association of County Behavioral Health and Developmental Disability Directors (NACBHDD). *The Challenge of Affordable Health Care: The ACA and Beyond*. Washington, DC.

Harrington, M. (1997). *The Other America*. New York: Scribner.

Kennedy Forum. (2016). *Navigating the New Frontier of Mental Health and Addiction: A Guide for the 115th Congress*. www.parityregistry.org; www.thekennedyforum.org; www.paritytrack.org.

Kennedy, P. J. (2015). *A Common Struggle: A Personal Journey through the Past and Future of Mental Illness and Addiction*. New York: Blue Rider Press.

Manderscheid, R. (March 23, 2015). *Stigma Kills: On the Five "P's" of Inclusion and Social Justice*. www.nacbhdd.org.

Manderscheid, R. (June 7, 2016). Helping rural counties keep abreast of urban counterparts. *Behavioral Healthcare Magazine*. www.behavioral.net.

Manderscheid, R. (August 28, 2016). Last chance to pass mental health reform? *Behavioral Healthcare Magazine*. www.behavioral.net.

Manderscheid, R. (August 30, 2016). *Hillary Clinton Offers Excellent Mental Health Policy Proposals*. www.behavioral.net.

Manderscheid, R. (December 19, 2016). *Treatment and Housing for Persons with Serious Mental Illness*. www.naco.org.

Mental Health America. (August 29, 2016). *Statement by Paul Gionfriddo, President and CEO, Mental Health America*. mhapostmaster@mentalhealthamerica.net

Mental Health and Rural America: 1994–2005. (2005). Washington, DC: Health Resources and Services Administration, Office of Rural Health Policy.

Mohatt, D. F. (2016). *Rural Mental Health: Challenges and Opportunities Caring for the Country*. Boulder, CO: Western Interstate Commission for Higher Education.

Morris, J. A. (1997). *Practicing Psychology in Rural Settings.* Washington, DC: American Psychological Association.

National Alliance on Mental Illness. (July 7, 2016). *We Did It! Mental Health Reform Is Headed to the President's Desk.* www.nami.org/About/NAMI/NAMI-news/We-Did-It-Mental-Health-Reform-Is-Headed-To-The-Presidents-Desk.

New Freedom Commission on Mental Health. (2003). A*chieving the Promise: Transforming Mental Health Care in America.* Final. DHHS Pub. Co. SMA-03-3832. Rockville, MD.

Quinn, M. (September, 2016). *Rural America Finally Gets Mental Health Help.* www.governing.com/templates/gov_print_article.

Redick, G. (January 5, 2016). *Obama's Executive Actions on Guns Draw Ire of Advocates for Mentally Ill.* Time Warner.

Rural Policy Research Institute. (2016). www.rupi.org.

Safran, M. A., Mays, R. A., Jr., Huang, L. N., McCuan, R., Pham, P. K., Fisher, S. K., McDuffie, K. Y., & Trachtenberg, A. (November, 2009). Mental health disparities. *American Journal of Public Health,* 99(11), 1962–1966.

Sawyer, D., Gale, J., & Lambert, D. (2006). *Rural and Frontier Mental and Behavioral Health Care: Barriers, Effective Policy Strategies, and Best Practices.* Washington, DC: National Association for Rural Mental Health.

Smalley, K. B., Warren, J., & Rainer, J. (Eds.). (2012). *Rural Mental Health: Issues, Policies, and Best Practices.* New York: Springer.

Smalley, K. B., Yancey, C. T., Warren, J. C., Naufel, K., Ryan, R., & Pugh, J. L. (2010). Rural mental health and psychological treatment: A review for practitioners. *Journal of Clinical Psychology: In Session,* 66(5), 479–489.

Smith, A. (2003). Rural mental health counseling: One example of practicing what the research preaches. *Journal of Rural Community Psychology,* E6(2), Fall.

Stamm, B. H. (Ed.). (2003). *Rural Behavioral Health Care.* Washington, DC: American Psychological Association.

Townsend, W. (2010). Recovery services in rural settings, strengths and challenges influencing behavioral healthcare service delivery. *Rural Mental Health,* 34(1), 23–32.

Vandiver, V. L. (2013). *Best Practices in Community Mental Health.* Chicago: Lyceum Books.

Weigel, D. (2009). *The Challenges of Rural Clinical Mental Health Counseling.* Weitz, Germany: VDM Verlag.

Whitaker, R. (2010). *Anatomy of an Epidemic.* New York: Broadway Books.

Wilson, W., Bangs, A., & Hatting, T. (February, 2015). *The Future of Rural Behavioral Health.* National Rural Health Association Policy Brief. www.ruralhealthnet.org.

Wood, R. E. (2008). *Survival of Rural America: Small Victories and Bitter Harvests.* Lawrence: University Press of Kansas.

3 Obstacles to Treatment— The Four "A's" and an "S"
Accessibility, Availability, Acceptability, Affordability, and Stigma

Although there is a similar prevalence of mental health issues in rural and urban areas, the obstacles to getting help are very different. This chapter explores the major obstacles to mental health treatment, which are accessibility, availability, acceptability, and affordability. Stigma is the largest barrier of all, as people in small communities are very hesitant to have others know that they are seeking outside help, preferring to cling to the stereotype of rugged individualism. The ratio of providers to residents is explored, as well as the issues surrounding the obstacles. The closing of psychiatric hospitals and workforce shortages are just two of the many barriers for rural populations to overcome in the quest for mental wellness.

What Are the Four A's, Their Implications, and Epidemiology?

The mental health system is a highly complicated quagmire of mumbo jumbo that, as a practitioner in the field, I still struggle to make sense of. We need a system that everyone can navigate clearly and easily. Currently, the mental health system in America is made up of a highly fragmented, elaborate group of public and private agencies that overlap to the point that it takes years to fully understand the way they operate individually and as a system. It's a classic example of the famous Abbott and Costello skit, "Who's on First?" Very often, public agencies contract with private agencies and the result is somewhat effective, depending on the geographic area. In Delaware County, New York, where I live, the Department of Social Services and the county mental health clinic are two separate entities, and the two don't communicate with each other enough. According to Stamm in *Rural Behavioral Health Care*, rural towns and communities have a unique opportunity to develop and maintain collaborative relationships because of the smaller number of stakeholders. He believes this should be the case across the spectrum of mental health providers and across the community's spectrum of health and human services, but sadly it is more the exception than the rule.

In general, there is equal prevalence of mental health issues in rural and urban communities. However, when rural residents are able to gain access to services, they often are required to accept compromises that include long-distance travel to receive care, limited choices of providers, loss of confidentiality as a result of the visibility of mental health services in small communities, and a heightened sense of personal stigma. This is all very discouraging to a person seeking help.

Many are the boulders rural folks have to climb over in order to obtain mental health services. Among the most common is the stigma mental health services have to people who, because of the isolated geography and the poor distribution of natural resources, have had to become rugged, self-sufficient individualists. Most people I know who have grown up in rural areas are far from the first generations to have internalized that kind of independent persona. As a society, we have romanticized that rugged individualism without realizing its costs. Mental illness causes more of the suffering in our society than physical illness, poverty, or unemployment do. It bars people on disability benefits, and accounts for nearly half of all days off sick. It affects educational achievement and income as much as pure IQ does.

We know that depression and anxiety alone account for more of the unhappiness in our country than physical illness does. Many believe they account for very much more unhappiness than is due to poverty or unemployment. So the front line in the fight against misery is the fight to get people to accept help.

The best predictor of whether or not a person would continue to suffer was the way they thought about and reacted to the trauma. Those with markedly negative thoughts and behavior continued to suffer while those whose thinking was more positive were much more likely to recover. The same is true of other forms of anxiety or depression, that those who recover are those who are least preoccupied with themselves. It is for this reason that volunteering is often recommended to people as an additional venue toward their own healing.

The four A's and an S have a highly complex relationship to each other, to the point that enhancing or fixing one area alone will not solve the problem. Solutions need to reach each of these areas in order to be successful.

Accessibility

The New Freedom Commission on Mental Health's Subcommittee on Rural Issues contends that one policy option is vital: rural Americans should be provided the same access to mental health emergency response, early identification and screening, diagnosis, treatment, and recovery services as their non-rural peers. The perception of a need for care is the first step in seeking care, and rural residents seem to enter care later than their urban peers due to their own lower perception of need. The problem is then compounded by rural residents perceiving that they have less access to care. Research shows that lower rates of access to mental health services are directly related to lower rates of availability of mental health providers.

30   *Obstacles to Treatment*

Rural populations exist in every state and territory in America. Geographic accessibility is a strong obstacle to rural families obtaining mental health services. Where I live, the nearest mental health clinic is a full hour ride away in good weather, as is the nearest crisis center (and they are in opposite directions). The price of gas notwithstanding, that is an unacceptable statistic in the 21st century. Currently in Delaware County, mental health practitioners have reached their capacity for number of clients, and people who see me as a private practitioner have to pay out of pocket because of antiquated state and federal regulations. The shortage of mental health practitioners would be less of a problem if more licensed, credentialed categories were allowed to take third party reimbursement, especially Medicaid.

A well-documented problem in rural areas—limited access to care—makes it necessary to be creative in restructuring the service delivery system, particularly for poor residents who are uninsured or underinsured. A solution that is being implemented slowly in rural areas is the integration of medical and mental health services in primary care offices. The result is being able to treat a person in a more holistic way; increased access to mental health services; decreased health care costs due to addressing physical, mental, and behavioral issues; and perhaps decreasing administrative costs by combining government-assisted Community Mental Health Centers and state departments of public health. This blending of physical and mental health is beginning to happen throughout the country, but it is a tediously slow process, and will take years before it becomes commonplace. In the meantime, there is little agreement of what integration of care looks like, how it should work, and what it will accomplish. That is not to mention the sometimes conflicting regulations each operates under. It would by necessity mean the integration of both providers and of procedures, and electronic files, of which there are many to consider.

My county was turned down for social workers at the Community Mental Health Center to be reimbursed for tuition if they work a set number of years at the clinic. This was because of a change in the formula for calculating need. The formula, based on a mixture of geographic variables, population groups, and types of facilities, designates shortage areas when the population-to-provider ratio exceeds certain thresholds. Because we are a very poor county, we are largely Medicaid reimbursed. The Community Mental Health Center in a neighboring community much less rural than Delaware County was approved for tuition reimbursement, as their rate of Medicaid reimbursement is much lower because being a less rural area, they have many more private practitioners.

Availability

According to the New Freedom Commission's Rural Subcommittee, the availability of rural mental health professionals depends on the complex blend of education, rural training opportunities, recruitment and retention activities, and continuing education and support. Rural America needs competent, dedicated professionals who have demonstrated knowledge and experience in rural/remote practice. The Rural Subcommittee believes that existing funding streams and training programs have missed the mark by not mandating a set of skills that would lead toward rural competency, developed in parallel with efforts toward establishing cultural and technical competency. This is among the reasons that rural areas are experiencing serious shortages of providers of mental and physical health services.

In my county in upstate New York, the ratio of mental health providers to residents is more than 950:1. The rest of the state averages 420:1.

The county departments of social services across the country need to update their antiquated methods of referral and payment for clients in need of therapy, especially in rural areas. Most of them will only hire professionals with an MSW, thereby eliminating any possibility of art therapists or any other kind of creative arts therapists working with and for them. Their referral systems have not been updated in decades, and they often shy away from providing access to therapy services at all. By not including mental health practitioners in their provider mix, their clients are losing out on the many benefits art and other therapies could provide.

My county mental health clinic, which serves many of its 48,000 people, has one part-time psychiatrist and a part-time psychiatric nurse practitioner to dole out psychotropic medication. The psychiatrist does not see children under the age of 12. The current trend of utilizing psychiatric nurse practitioners (PNPs) has helped ease the waiting lists for mental health services to some degree, but many more are needed in order for rural residents' medication needs to be met. This trend is not only more cost-effective, but it has often been my experience that PNPs have a better understanding of rural culture and are more committed to remaining in a rural area.

The closing of many psychiatric hospitals across the country created even larger barricades to availability of mental health services in rural areas. In 2013, New York State Senator Tom Libous proposed legislation to freeze the closures of numerous psychiatric hospitals in his state, including one that is 2 hours from my town and the closest psychiatric hospital besides Albany. He saw that these facilities provide essential inpatient services to individuals with serious mental illness or with intellectual and other developmental disabilities, including many who are frail, dangerous, or violent. He also saw that because of these hospital closures, families would have to travel hours to visit their loved ones getting inpatient care. In addition, individuals who may not be ready for community living will be pushed out the hospital door without any adequate planning for local alternatives. He felt it would be cutting the safety net for the most fragile members of our rural communities. The closing of these facilities could also force state employees to seek new jobs and move to new communities. The psychiatric hospital closures also mean overcrowded hospital emergency rooms and inundated local correctional facilities. Those scenarios shift the cost rather than eliminate or reduce it. According to a source from the county mental health clinic, Delaware

County has approximately 100 admissions per year to the Binghamton Psychiatric Hospital. Three adolescents from my town alone were admitted there last year. Their families were able to get gas vouchers to help offset the high cost of gasoline last year in order to visit their loved ones who were over two hours away. The hospital would have been closed had it not been for the legislature's intervention.

Other trends made available through advances in technology, such as telemedicine, are slowly reaching rural areas, but much more is needed in order to have ample access to qualified mental health providers. And let's face it: there is no substitute for honest-to-goodness, face-to-face contact. This solution is a mixed blessing because it cuts down on travel time and expense but maintains the distance from human contact for people, many of whom are already geographically isolated.

In addition, many rural farm workers and other types of non-permanent full-time workers, and people who have part-time jobs or seasonal employment, do not have any medical benefits at all, nor can they afford to pay anything out of pocket. Hopefully the Affordable Care Act will remedy that problem.

Many believe that those of us who work in the mental health field approach their jobs and practices as if they are a business. In a sense they are businesses, but without the warmth and safety a caring practitioner provides, no real growth takes place. Those of my peers who approach their practices competitively are clearly in the "business" of making money with less concern for the well-being of their clients. Competition is unconscionable and unnecessary in the mental health field. Many believe that we should consider and market ourselves as a part of the greater health care industry, and indeed with the increasing mandates to link to primary care facilities, we will also be physically tied to the health care industry. The laws and regulations, however, need to follow suit and reflect that link in order to allow it to work properly.

Rural Mental Health Realities

- The number of psychiatrists in urban areas: 14.6 per 100,000
- The number of psychiatrists in rural areas: 3.9 per 100,000
- More than 85% of 1,669 federally designated mental health professional shortage areas are rural.

(Bird, Dempsey, and Hartley, 2001)

Acceptability

It is well known that rural residents tend to value self-reliance and view seeking help in more negative ways than urban residents. For many, it boils down to feeling it totally unacceptable to be seen in the waiting room of a mental health clinic or for anyone to see their car parked like a flag outside the office. The National Association for Rural Mental Health (NARMH) reported that the social stigma of mental illness, lack of rural-specific technical assistance, mistrust of health professionals in some rural and frontier communities, and lack of cultural competence in spite of increasing diversity are the top barriers and concerns regarding mental health service delivery in rural America.

The NARMH also reported financing issues that create barriers to acceptable mental health service. They include uncertainty of public funding streams, lack of flexible funding streams, lack of funding for prescription medication, complicated and cumbersome funding arrangements, restrictive reimbursements, lack of funding for evidence-based practices specifically for rural areas, reimbursement issues with telehealth services, complex funding systems that are fragmented and lead to increased costs for providers, higher cost of service delivery in rural areas due to low volume of patients and managed care organizations placing unnecessary restrictions on provider types, and lack of insurance coverage for mental and behavioral health services or higher premiums or co-pays compared to other physical illnesses, are all just a few of the issues forming a barrier to acceptability in mental health care, particularly in rural areas.

There are many structural and organizational issues that create barriers to acceptability in care as well. According to the NARMH, a few of the contributing barriers are insufficient communication among primary care providers and Community Mental Health Centers, incompatible software and hardware and inadequate infrastructure for telehealth connections, limited availability of clinicians with prescriptive authority, lack of specialists, especially those with child/adolescent expertise. Other logistic barriers include lack of public transportation, distances and difficulties accessing care even when private transportation is available, lack of coordination among federal agencies, especially the Health Resources and Services Administration (HRSA) and the Substance Abuse and Mental Health Services Administration (SAMHSA). The need for practitioners to be generalists and the lack of integration of mental health with primary care and substance abuse services in many areas add to the difficulties faced by rural providers when competing for funding. Lack of organizational capacity or expertise, or the use of urban criteria for contracts in calculating required credentialed professional staff by government agencies, lack of support for affordable housing, comprehensive rehabilitation programs, peer support services, comprehensive needs assessment data specific to rural and frontier areas, the unintended impact of federal regulations such as the Health Insurance Portability and Accountability Act of 1996 (HIPAA), and the unaddressed behavioral health care needs of rural women and many children round out the list of barriers to acceptable mental health care.

The NARMH lists the main workforce barriers to good mental services in many rural areas. They include lack of trained staff members/providers/clinicians, lack of adequate professionals to treat dual diagnoses, lack of telehealth services, lack of continuing educational opportunities (in my case, the state requires presenters to pay $900 to be able to grant continuing education credits to Licensed Creative Arts Therapists (LCATs), and they have increased the number of continuing education units required in order to maintain licensing), excessive waiting lists for services, lack of financial incentives for professionals to work in rural areas (think tuition reimbursement, increased vacation time, perhaps bonuses), lack of scholarships and grants for training, poor dissemination of training information to rural practitioners, and inadequate health and prescription drug benefits—especially for those who are self-employed. I would add to this list lack of funding for research into rural mental health populations and their issues.

Finally, the NARMH suggests ways that state Offices of Rural Health as well as other agencies can help. They state,

> There is hope that state Offices of Rural Health can become a driving force behind developing networks and collaborations of relevant organizations to improve services and increase patient access. State Offices of Rural Health are essential partners, bridging primary care and mental health systems together, targeting program delivery to specific databased state and local needs, and encouraging collaborative partnerships. They are important in identifying and establishing linkages with underserved populations and connecting local peer-type programs with state and federal systems for such underserved groups. They can be helpful in partnering the administration and delivery of rural services, especially in pilot and model programs where delivery skills are high but administrative and general management skills may be lacking. Finally, they can be an essential player in information and model sharing at both the state and regional levels.

Authors Sawyer, Gale, and Lambert stated in their 2006 NARMH report that state and national policy makers continue to operate under a consistent and pervasive misunderstanding of rural realities. As a result, they do not adequately account for these rural realities when developing public policy and they continue to seek a single policy solution to rural issues rather than combine ideas and have agencies do more collaborating.

Affordability

Medicare reimbursement rates are often lower in rural areas. The farm bill of 1987 included the Rural Crisis Recovery Act, which helped support direct funding of rural health services. Community efforts such as these are often limited by the lack of long-term funding to ensure sustainability. In my own area, the local hospital secured a 1-year grant to pay a psychiatrist to work with children 2 days a week. The idea was that children with medication needs would have local access to someone with expertise in dealing with children and adolescents. It all worked out fine—until the funds ran out 9 months into the program. By that point, many children had nowhere to turn to continue their psychotropic medications but their primary care physicians, assuming they had one, and their therapeutic alliance with the provider was severed rather abruptly. Government grants such as the one we received locally ought to be issued for multiple years and while providing help to local grantees in planning for sustainability and measuring results.

In *The Survival of Rural America*, Wood laments that rural America is unlikely ever to be able to force the country to pay attention to it. Congress prefers to address rural issues, including those that have little or nothing to do with farming, within the context of its omnibus 5-year farm bills, and it has been reluctant to accept proposals that don't fit within the farm bill framework. They have in effect connected rural and agricultural policy by using public dollars to funnel into agriculture with the idea that if agriculture does well, rural would do well by extension. They don't see that these are two separate issues.

Wood continues to explain that federal farm policy can be divided into two distinct eras: before and after 1933. Prior to 1933, the federal government's involvement in farmers' finances consisted primarily of monetary controls. Although the United States was originally an agrarian economy, the US Department of Agriculture (USDA) was not even created until 1962 and did not achieve cabinet status until 1989. Today we grow about three times as much food on one-third of the land, using just two-thirds of the manpower, as we did before World War II.

The gist of public policy complaints seems to be the contention that federal subsidy programs favor large farmers at the expense of small ones. The complaint has merit. According to the Kellogg Foundation, the largest federal rural program by far is the farm subsidy program. The charge that most of this subsidy goes to large farmers and to corporate or industrial farms would appear to be borne out by the finding that more than 60% of federal farm subsidy payments go to just 7.2% of the farmers participating in the program. The Kellogg report points out another problem with federal policies: although about 90% of rural income is derived from non-farming sources, and agriculture only accounts for about 6% of rural employment, much more federal support goes to farming subsidies than to rural business and community development efforts, which would benefit a far larger percentage of people living in rural America.

In 2006 the USDA's total budget was just under $95 billion, of which only 2% went for rural development. However, if rural development is measured as a part of what the USDA considers its discretionary budget of $20 billion, the share increases to about 10%. The big—and in many cases nondiscretionary—items in the USDA budget were, and are likely to remain, food and nutrition (58%), which includes food stamps and childhood nutrition programs, and the Farm Service Agency (30%), which handles loans and income-support payments to farmers. And some federal dollars also find their way to rural America through other government departments, including Housing and Urban Development, Health and Human Services, the Department of Transportation, the Department of Education, the Department of Commerce, and others.

Many view the 2007 farm bill as a tweaking of the prior bill, keeping expenditures for rural development and other programs over the next 5 years close to 2002 levels. Specific rural programs in the 2007 bill include $1.6 billion in guaranteed loans to complete the rehabilitation of more than 1,200 rural Critical Access Hospitals and $500 million for rural infrastructure projects such as water, waste disposal, and telecommunications. The infrastructure funding in the 2007 farm bill is similar to some portions of the Rural Renaissance Act, although amounts proposed are smaller. The 2007 bill did not adopt the approach of the New Homestead Act of specifically trying to attract people to depopulating rural areas. It did, however, propose an important program designed to provide additional support for farmers and ranchers who are starting out, recognizing the high cost of purchasing farm land and capital equipment and taking into consideration the average age of the current generation of farmers. The federal program would supplement several existing smaller-scale efforts to help new farmers that are offered through some of the land-grant universities and the Farm Beginnings program of the nonprofit Land Stewardship Project, which offers courses and mentoring programs. The 2007 farm bill stalled late in the year due to differences in outlook among Congress members, on subjects such as conservation, rural development, and budgeting and commodity support policy. The deadlock increased the likelihood that the 2007 bill would emerge with few major differences from the 2002 bill.

The Clinton Health Care Act died in 1994, and with it any chances for mental illness and treatment for people with addictions to be an equal part of the larger health care reform package. At this point in time, people with preexisting conditions were usually denied coverage, and lifetime caps dictated how much money a citizen could use toward their physical and mental health over their lifetime. At that time, parity seemed like a pretty basic concept that turned out to be anything but. Among the largest issues were exactly what would and would not be covered by a parity law, and how parity could be created and enforced. Would parity cover all mental illnesses, which in theory included any condition listed in the DSM (the *Diagnostic and Statistical Manual*, the "bible" of mental health professionals)? Would parity also include all treatment for people with addictions and substance use disorders?

Patrick Kennedy wanted parity to cover a menu of evidence-based treatments from different caregivers in different settings that worked for different patients—the equivalent of covering surgery, medication, outpatient physical therapy, inpatient rehab, and other treatments for a knee injury, not merely generic psychopharmacology, a little short-term outpatient therapy, and maybe a few days in a hospital after a suicide attempt. He, like many others, felt that this was unacceptable mental health treatment. The parity bill was designed to fix the disparities that were increasing and gaining attention. According to the *American Journal of Public Health*, mental health disparities are complex, challenging problems that involve multiple determining factors at the individual, community, program, system, and policy levels. They present a special challenge to government because they defy definition, cut across policy and service areas, and often resist solutions offered by the single-agency approach.

And what would parity actually mean, once the law got beyond banning the denial of coverage based on pre-existing conditions, unequal co-pays and lifetime caps for mental health care? How would the parity law remedy problems like the shortages of qualified caregivers in various parts of the country, and shortages of mental health beds and facilities for inpatient and outpatient care? If mental health care merged with traditional medicine, what kind of law would insure that the transition was smooth and continued to work in a patient's best interest?

And would any of these changes actually lessen the stigma of mental health diagnoses and mental health care to the point where most of the people who needed help would get it and participate in treatment as long as needed?

At least the Iowa caucuses, the starting point of the presidential primaries, forces candidates to focus on rural issues, however briefly, every 4 years. The second presidential primary happens in New Hampshire, another state that is almost entirely rural, where voters during the 2016 primaries raised rural issues with presidential candidates. Heroin is a particularly huge problem in New Hampshire, bringing the issue further into the national spotlight.

During the summer of 2011, President Obama established the White House Rural Council by Executive Order #13575, naming access to affordable health care among the council's top priorities. He established the council knowing that about 20% of the American population lives in rural communities, and that strong, sustainable rural communities are essential to ensuring American competitiveness in the years ahead. Obama believed that because rural communities supply our food, fiber, and energy, safeguard our natural resources, are essential in the development of science and innovation, and face numerous economic challenges, they also present enormous economic potential. He believed that the federal government plays an important role in expanding access to the capital necessary for economic growth, promoting innovation, improving access to health care and education, and expanding outdoor recreational activities on public lands. He created the council in order to enhance the federal government's efforts to address the needs of rural America and dedicate an investment in rural communities throughout the country in order to promote the economic prosperity and quality of life in these small communities. The council was charged with coordinating and increasing the effectiveness of federal engagement with rural stakeholders, providers, telecommunications services providers, research and land grant institutions, law enforcement, state, local and tribal governments, and non-governmental organizations regarding the needs of rural America.

Rural policy will be increasingly affected by environmental issues such as energy, water, and the need to preserve rural areas as the reserve for urban areas rather than places that deserve development in their own right. Residents of my area have for decades been pressured mercilessly and economically suffocated by the powers governing the New York City water commission, and they have successfully limited economic development in our area by imposing

38   Obstacles to Treatment

stringent restrictions on the types of industries and businesses that can legally operate within their designated watershed area. Thus, the economic development in this rural mountainous region is further stunted.

In the United States, we view trade and commodity policy as being on the national level, while we view services and infrastructure on the state level, and economic development and services at the local level. Rural development is seen as a local initiative. Yet the New York City water restrictions have severely limited most kinds of economic development in a series of counties among the poorest in the state. Delaware County alone houses two of the main reservoirs built and used by the city of New York. In order to build these reservoirs, whole towns were deserted and bulldozed so that the lowlands could be flooded. Thousands of families were forced to leave their homes, their land and their community, and relocate wherever they could afford to.

The "S" Word: Stigma—Its Causes and Implications in Rural Areas

According to Ron Manderscheid, "Stigma Kills." The director of the National Association of County Behavioral Health and Developmental Disability Directors (NACBHDD) addressed the issue of stigma by explaining that people with mental health and substance abuse conditions die an average of 25 years before others without those conditions. In addition, it takes an average of a decade before most rural people access the treatment they need. Suicide rates remain high throughout America while death rates due to substance abuse continue to rise. So what keeps people from seeking help until their psychic pain has become severe enough that they have turned into a complex mix of somatic and psychological disabilities? Some liken this to a cancer patient seeking treatment when they reach stage 4 of their illness.

Stigma consists of many facets, including stereotypes, prejudice, judgment, and discrimination. There is stigma generated from the outside inward, and self-stigma, which is generated from the inside radiating outward. Self-stigma happens when individuals internalize public stigma by accepting and applying negative stereotypes to themselves. Individuals experiencing self-stigma often have low self-esteem, often poor quality social interactions, diminished relationships, and increased unemployment.

How can policy reduce stigmatization that prevents people from accessing care, living successfully in the community, and sustaining recovery? Manderscheid advocates for a 5-point reform plan that includes:

- *Parity*: Parity changes are not fully applicable to Medicaid and Medicare recipients in most states, further exacerbating stigma for people and families experiencing poverty. In order to reach true parity, we need to extend it to equal housing, equal jobs, equal supports, and equal pay.
- *Practice*: The system is moving toward fully integrated care through team-based practice approaches and integrated funding models. True practice integration must integrate behavioral health clients with all other

clients in health and medical homes. Stigmatization can sustain practices of exclusion that separate people with behavioral health needs out and away from their peers and people experiencing other health-related concerns. "Separate but equal" cannot remain a valid practice strategy if our system aims to achieve parity.

- *Promotion*: The ACA emphasizes using resources toward health promotion and prevention. Activities that sustain these opportunities are also ones that can pay for resources in the community that help clients recover, experience wellness, and live full lives. Promoting recovery through policy means that states and counties need to swiftly invest in integrated practice that promotes and rewards early intervention and wellness-based strategies. These types of services have been minimally financed since psychiatric hospitals started closing decades ago. Integrating these services into mainstream financing mechanisms and incorporating them into discharge planning and whole-health treatment plans is essential to promoting community recovery.
- *Peers*: Developing a peer workforce can only enhance parity reforms and promote dignity and community-based recovery. People with lived experience can actively reduce stigmatization by gaining employment, and helping consumers and family members understand that behavioral health is not something to be feared or diminished. Peers should work across the health system, not just with behavioral health clients, to offer a wide range of experiences, values, and capacity to people in recovery across the wellness spectrum.
- *Participation*: Moving "out of the office" toward inclusive participation doesn't only include outreach and engagement in services. Participative, community-based action includes public demonstrations, legislative hearings, key meetings with public leaders and executives, and coalition building among organizational leaders. Raising the visibility of a recovery-based movement is essential to reducing the stigma associated with mental health and substance abuse treatment.
- In conclusion, Manderscheid says that if we begin with a human rights-based approach to equality, and capitalize on the gains made in the ACA, we can achieve measurable reductions in stigmatization through incorporation of the steps outlined above. Defeating stigma demands civil rights and social justice actions at every level, including transparency of effective policy leadership in state and local governments. We are all responsible for reducing stigma, and we can all create opportunities for growth and change from policy to practice.

Adding to stigma is the location of the mental health clinic or therapist's office. When everyone in town knows your car and it is parked at a mental health office, it sits like a flag waving your name. In my private practice, I don't hang a shingle out front on purpose. This way it is difficult to distinguish why someone might be parked there. This has been an issue in urban and rural areas and will continue to be until stigma regarding mental health shrinks.

Rural Matters: The Memorial Day Parade

The Memorial Day float holds the broken dreams of every dead soldier's family. It glides behind the firemen's drum and bugle corps; the bass drum is the heartbeat of the parade. Those regal men and women in uniform march to the bullet-like beats as spectators cheer. Anyone not marching lines Main Street—some standing, others in yard chairs, some with dogs, others with babies and grandparents. Everyone knows everyone else. Those who parade are neighbors and friends, bosses, co-workers, or acquaintances. Those of us watching are all that is left. I wonder if there are more paraders than spectators.

Between marching groups are the town's fire trucks and ambulances driven by friends and neighbors, even our school superintendent, who is an emergency medical technician. American flags are draped on every telephone pole for this occasion, as they are draped on every coffin of every soldier who is killed. Many who are killed are from rural areas like this. A disproportionate percentage of rural young people join the military. It's always been that way. We all know families whose lives were shattered in one way or another by the loss of a loved one in war times or lives disrupted.

This parade always makes me teary-eyed. I feel it especially this year, as some of the kids I've watched grow up since they were very young are joining the military. Three of them out of a graduating class of 28. They grew up with my daughter. For some, it's their only ticket out of this small, provincial town. For others, it's been their dream for many years. And for still others, it just came about by a series of coincidences. For all, they will put themselves in harm's way to protect the rest of us. It's so hard to watch them go.

The parade follows with the high school marching band, which consists of a dozen students doing their best to play from their patriotic hearts. Then follow Girl Scouts of all ages and the Cub and Boy Scouts, all wearing uniforms and carrying banners. We smile and wave to them all as they go by and they wave back sneaking a look askance before returning to look straight ahead. To some we throw kisses. It's a small world we live in here. For me, the wonder of the parade is that small world and the ways we are all intertwined like trees in the forest. Kids on floats throw candy to those of us lining the street. As parents we always knew where to position our child and her friends so they would be sure to collect optimal amounts of candy from the pavement as the floats coast by. My daughter would shout so excitedly, "Oh here are some Tootsie Rolls, and oh, there are some Snickers Bars, my favorite." And so it went until all of our pockets overflowed with sugary treats.

One year I marched in the parade as the Daisy leader of my daughter's troop. We had a grand time waving and throwing candy to the sparse crowd lining the street, always sure to throw some directly to the youngsters we knew. Just recovering from a broken ankle, I hobbled down Main Street with my crutches. I must have looked hysterical. When she was slightly older, my daughter rode in the back of a pickup truck with her fellow Girl Scouts, as proud of her candy-throwing self as we were of her. She waved with the other girls to those of us lining the streets, being sure to yell, "Hi mom and dad," as she passed by the corner of our street. "This is for you, Fudgie," she yelled to our dog as we tried to keep him from eating the candy strewn along the pavement.

When the large fire trucks began to coast by, we all felt a special wave of gratitude and pride. Spectators clapping, cheering, and whistling temporarily drowned out all other sound. Aside from the usual firefighting and emergency ambulance runs they performed, they had many other chances to show their excellence. They performed many rescues, as did the ambulance, during Hurricane Irene, when this area was utterly flooded and laden with wind damage. Many people in the surrounding countryside needed to be rescued from their homes as the flood waters rose quicker than we could ever imagine. Our dear friends were delivered to us that stormy morning from the back of an ambulance that appeared at their house just in the nick of time before the rising water made the road impassable. Moments later, it pulled up in front of our house, and out they came from the back of the ambulance, one by one climbing down the back step onto the puddled street and running up the driveway and into our small, dry house. It was their fourth time being flooded. They lived in a flat valley that seemed to catch more than the average amount of rainfall. Eventually their house was bought out with flood recovery funds and knocked down. The only sign that it ever existed is a tree that they planted in memory of their son who had died several years earlier.

They are all volunteers, the firemen, emergency medical technicians, and the auxiliary members who support them. They have regular jobs and families, and some even farm obligations to fulfill even if they are called out on an emergency. Some high school students train to join the firemen, and stay with it through adulthood. Many are the subzero nights the fire alarm goes off during the wee hours, or on the hottest muggiest days, days of torrential rain, icy roads and blizzards. Nothing stops them. They consider it their civic duty.

This year the parade topped out at 20 minutes. Afterward, community members congregate at the town green, where there is a short tribute to our fallen soldiers and a gun salute. Dogs cower throughout town and birds freeze in their tracks. Many like us linger on street corners talking with friends and neighbors, some we haven't seen since before the long winter.

The firemen leave soon after for other parades, showing off our shiny equipment in the spring sunlight of other small towns. For the rest of the day and then some, I am filled with the wonder of living in a small community and with the gratitude I have for those men and women in different kinds of uniforms. There is just nothing else like these small-town community events to remind us of what is truly important.

References

Bagalman, E. (2016). *The Helping Families in Mental Health Crisis Reform Act of 2016*. Washington, DC: Congressional Research Service.

Berg-Cross, L., Reviere, R., Miller, J., Chappell, A., & Salmon, A. (2001). Certification of mental health advocates: A call to action. *Journal of Rural Community Psychology*, E14(1).

Bird, D.C., Dempsey, P., & Hartley, D. (2001). *Efforts to Address Mental Health Workforce Needs in Underserved Rural Areas.* University of Southern Maine, Institute for Health Policy, Maine Rural Health Research Center (Working Paper #23).

Brown, D., & Swanson, L. (Eds.). (2003). *Challenges for Rural America in the Twenty-First Century.* University Park: Pennsylvania State University Press.

Carter, R. (2010). *Within Our Reach: Ending the Mental Health Crisis.* Emmaus, PA: Rodale Books.

Cloke, P., Marsden, T., & Mooney, P. H. (Eds.). (2006). *Handbook of Rural Studies.* Thousand Oaks, CA: Sage.

Coalition for Mental Health Reform (CMHR). (July 6, 2016). *Concerns With the Helping Families in Mental Health: Crisis Act of 2015—Passed in the House of Representatives.*

County Health Rankings and Roadmaps (CHRR). *A Robert Wood Johnson Foundation Program.* www.countyhealthrankings.org.

Elder, G., & Conger, R. (Eds.). (2000). *Children of the Land: Adversity and Success in Rural America.* Chicago: University of Chicago Press.

Federal Office of Rural Health Policy (FORHP) (April 5, 2017). *FORHP Announcements: What's New.* Washington, DC.

Gladding, S.T. (1997). *Community and Agency Counseling.* Upper Saddle River, NJ: Prentice-Hall.

Goldman, H.H., Buck, J.A., & Thompson, K.S. (2009). *Transforming Mental Health Services: Implementing the Federal Agenda for Change.* Arlington, VA: American Psychiatric Association.

Grantham, D. (February 1, 2017). National Association of County Behavioral Health and Developmental Disability Directors (NACBHDD). *The Challenge of Affordable Health Care: The ACA and Beyond.* Washington, DC.

Group for the Advancement of Psychiatry. (1995). *Mental Health in Remote Rural Developing Areas.* Washington, DC: American Psychiatric Press.

Hartley. D., Bird, D., Lambert, D., & Coffin, J. (November, 2002). *The Role of Community Mental Health Centers as Rural Safety Net Providers.* Portland: University of Southern Maine, Edmund S. Muskie School of Public Service, Maine Rural Health Research Center (Working Paper #30).

Imhoff, D. (2012). *Food Fight: The Citizens Guide to the Next Food and Farm Bill.* Healdsburg, CA: Watershed Media.

Kagan, R., & Schlosberg, S. (1989). *Families in Perpetual Crisis.* New York: W.W. Norton.

Layard, R., & Clark, D. (2015). *Thrive: How Better Mental Health Care Transforms Lives and Saves Money.* Princeton, NJ: Princeton University Press.

Manderscheid, R. (March 23, 2015). *Stigma Kills: On the Five "P's" of Inclusion and Social Justice.* www.nacbhdd.org.

Obama, B. (June 9, 2011). *Establishment of the White House Rural Council, Executive Order* #13575. Washington, DC: Office of the Federal Register. www.hsdl.org.

President's New Freedom Commission on Mental Health. (May 5, 2002). Washington, DC: Executive Office of the President. pp. 22337–22338.

Sawyer, D., Gale, J., & Lambert, D. (2006). *Rural and Frontier Mental and Behavioral Health Care: Barriers, Effective Policy Strategies, and Best Practices.* Washington, DC: National Association for Rural Mental Health.

Smalley, K.B., Yancey, C.T., Warren, J.C., Naufel, K., Ryan, R., & Pugh, J.L. (2010). Rural mental health and psychological treatment: A review for practitioners. *Journal of Clinical Psychology: In Session*, 66(5), 479–489.

Stamm, B.H. (Ed.). (2003). *Rural Behavioral Health Care.* Washington, DC: American Psychological Association.

Wood, R. E. (2008). *Survival of Rural America: Small Victories and Bitter Harvests.* Lawrence: University Press of Kansas.

4 The Structure of Rural Mental Health Care
State, County, Town, Village

This chapter explores the structure of rural mental health care on the local level. It looks at the effects of urbanormative thinking on rural life, the structure of rural local governments, the origin and purpose of the Community Services Board (CSB) on the county level, as well as the origin and goals of the Community Mental Health Clinics (CMHC).

Most rural counseling programs are created as scaled-down versions of an urban model in spite of the fact that research shows that the mental health needs of rural Americans are separate and different from those in urban areas. Studies show that rural residents go for longer periods of time without insurance than urban residents and therefore have a greater likelihood of pent-up issues. In addition, they are more likely not to seek physician services when they cannot pay, both because of pride and limited opportunities for free or reduced-fee clinical care. Lack of insurance can be especially tragic for families with children with serious emotional disturbances (SEDs). Parents should never have to face the unthinkable choice of relinquishing custody of their child to obtain mental health treatment because they cannot pay for care. And yet it happens.

The Structure of Local Governments

Local decision-makers struggle with how to transform fragmented care into coordinated service delivery systems. For the most part, specialty practices are not lucrative enough to sustain themselves in rural areas. And because there is a great deal of diversity between rural areas across the country, services in a given area will have more successful results if providers understand the unique history and qualities of a given community. In a great many rural towns, there is no mayor, but rather a town supervisor. A town supervisor functions in very much the same way as a mayor would, but it is a part-time position, and a generally low paid one at that. At the county level, many rural counties are governed by a board of supervisors, made up of each town supervisor or mayor within the county boundaries. It is their job to oversee the general business of the county, including the mental health clinic, the commissioner of social services, and all other county organizations within its jurisdiction. Therefore, the director of community mental health services reports to the Community Services Board and, ultimately, the county board of supervisors. What is not clear is how many of the issues these boards face are taken to the state level, where there is potential for help and potentially even financial aid. If our state legislators and officials don't know about the issues, they can't be of help.

A Cornell University research report from 2010 states that rural residents consider their local officials and local to be accessible and responsive to their needs. In contrast, they consider state agencies to be unresponsive. Some of the characteristics that rural constituents see as local government strengths may also be their weaknesses. For example, local governments are small in size, which may increase efficiency and reactivity to local issues; it may also reduce efficiency through lack of local accountability. Regional collaboration and intermunicipal resource sharing increase efficiency and effectiveness. Limited competition for public offices is another challenge for local governments and communities. Public officials in rural areas are generally part-time employees with other jobs and responsibilities, and the turnover rate can be high due to lack of incentives, becoming tangled in local controversies while living in their communities, inadequate training, lack of funding and applicability for state mandates that are often urbancentric, local resistance to change, lack of regional cohesion and willingness to partner on projects and resources.

The Community Services Board (CSB)

The Community Mental Health Centers Act of 1963 (with amendments in 1975 and 1977), created accessible clinics responsible for a wide range of services, including inpatient, outpatient, consultation, education, evaluation and assessment, and crisis intervention. It was created to link these clinics directly to the community and to other community agencies such as departments of social services, probation, law enforcement, and drug and alcohol services. Members of the community at large with a marked interested in mental health issues serve on the committee as volunteer board members, hopefully representing many different points of view. This includes a town supervisor to represent the county board of supervisors.

Generally, the CSB's purpose is to maintain a program of comprehensive mental health services that are required for the treatment, habilitation, and rehabilitation of the county residents it represents. Included under the category of mental health services are treatment and prevention of mental illness for residents of all ages, mental health education, alcoholism and substance abuse treatment, and services for people with developmental disabilities.

On a funding and regulatory level, community mental health clinics report to their state department of mental health; when dealing with local issues, they report to the board of supervisors of their county.

In the time I served on my local CSB, I learned a great deal about how local mental health clinics operate, the issues they face, as well as the population they serve. It was an eye-opening experience, one completely different from being a mental health practitioner.

Community Mental Health Centers (CMHC)

The 1963 Community Mental Health Centers Act and its amendments marked the birth of the CMHC concept. President Kennedy signed the bill into law just 3 weeks before he was assassinated. The bill, which was revolutionary for its time, required counties to create CMHCs and provide five core elements of services to community members: outpatient, inpatient, consultation/education, partial hospitalization, and emergency/crisis intervention. Kennedy ensured that all community members would be served regardless of their ability to pay for the services. In rural areas, CMHCs were the only game in town offering sliding fee payment scales.

In part as a consequence of the deinstitutionalization movement that began in the 1960s, many CMHCs were forced to abandon their role as multipurpose service agencies in order to devote an increasing share of their resources to the needs of individuals defined by their state mental health agencies as members of priority populations. For the most part, these populations were identified as either children under the age of 18 with a serious emotional disturbance who exhibit severe emotional or social disabilities that are life threatening or require prolonged intervention, or adults with severe and persistent mental illness such as schizophrenia, major depression, bipolar disorder, or other severely disabling mental disorders that require crisis resolution or ongoing support and treatment.

References

Alliance for Health Reform (AHR). *Essentials of Health Policy: A Sourcebook for Journalists and Policymakers.* www.sourcebook.allhealth.org.

Brown, D. L., & Schafft, K. (2011). *Rural People and Communities.* Malden, MA: Polity Press.

Butler, C., Butler, J., & Gasteyer, S. (2016). *Rural Communities: Legacy and Change* (5th ed.). Boulder, CO: Westview Press.

Castle, E. (Ed.). (1995). *The Changing American Countryside: Rural People and Places.* Lawrence: University Press of Kansas.

Census.gov/geo/tiger/glossary2.html.

Childs, A. W., & Melton, G. B. (1983). *Rural Psychology.* New York: Plenum Press.

Cloke, P., Marsden, T., & Mooney, P. H. (Eds.). (2006). *Handbook of Rural Studies.* Thousand Oaks, CA: Sage.

Coalition for Mental Health Reform (CMHR). (July 6, 2016). *Concerns With the Helping Families in Mental Health: Crisis Act of 2015—Passed in the House of Representatives.*

Cornell University. (2010). *Poverty, Local and Regional Government, Energy, Economic and Workforce Development, Agriculture and Food Systems.* Ithaca, NY. www.cornell.edu.

Danbom, D. H. (2006). *Born in the Country: A History of Rural America.* Baltimore: Johns Hopkins University Press.

Federal Office of Rural Health Policy (FORHP). (April 5, 2017). *FORHP Announcements: What's New*. Washington, DC.

Flora, C.B., & Flora, J.L. (2008). *Rural Communities, Legacy and Change* (3rd ed.). Philadelphia, PA: Westview Press/Perseus Books.

Ginsberg, L.H. (2005). *Social Work in Rural Communities* (4th ed.). Alexandria, VA: Council on Social Work Education.

Gladding, S.T. (1997). *Community and Agency Counseling*. Upper Saddle River, NJ: Prentice-Hall.

Goldman, H.H., Buck, J.A., & Thompson, K.S. (2009). *Transforming Mental Health Services: Implementing the Federal Agenda for Change*. Arlington, VA: American Psychiatric Association.

Grantham, D. (April 1, 2016). National Association of County Behavioral Health and Developmental Disability Directors (NACBHDD). *Under the Microscope: Salt Lake County's System of Care Thrives in Hostile Funding Environment*. Washington, DC.

Grantham, D. (February 1, 2017). National Association of County Behavioral Health and Developmental Disability Directors (NACBHDD). *The Challenge of Affordable Health Care: The ACA and Beyond*. Washington, DC.

Grantham, D. (June 1, 2015). National Association of County Behavioral Health and Developmental Disability Directors (NACBHDD). *Under the Microscope: Developing Effective Alternatives to Incarceration for Those With MH and SUD Conditions*. Washington, DC.

Group for the Advancement of Psychiatry. (1995). *Mental Health in Remote Rural Developing Areas*. Washington, DC: American Psychiatric Press.

Hartley, D., Bird, D., Lambert, D., & Coffin, J. (November, 2002). *The Role of Community Mental Health Centers as Rural Safety Net Providers*. Portland: University of Southern Maine, Edmund S. Muskie School of Public Service, Maine Rural Health Research Center (Working Paper #30).

Hartley, D., Ziller, E., Lambert, D., Loux, S., & Bird, D. (October, 2002). *State Licensure Laws and the Mental Health Professions: Implications for the Rural Mental Health Workforce*. Portland: University of Southern Maine, Edmund S. Muskie School of Public Service, Maine Rural Health Research Center (Working Paper #29).

Imhoff, D. (2012). *Food Fight: The Citizens Guide to the Next Food and Farm Bill*. Healdsburg, CA: Watershed Media.

Kennedy, J.F. (October 31, 1963). *Remarks on Signing Mental Retardation Facilities and Community Health Centers Construction Bill* (Speech). Signing S. 1576, the Community Presidential Library and Museum. JFKPOF-047-045.

Manderscheid, R. (June 7, 2016). Helping rural communities keep abreast of urban counterparts. *Behavioral Healthcare Magazine*. www.behavioral.net.

Mental Health America. (August 29, 2016). *Statement by Paul Gionfriddo, President and CEO, Mental Health America*. mhapostmaster@mentalhealthamerica.net.

Mental Health and Rural America: 1994–2005. (2005). Washington, DC: Health Resources and Services Administration, Office of Rural Health Policy.

New Freedom Commission on Mental Health. (2003). *Achieving the Promise: Transforming Mental Health Care in America*. Final. DHHS Pub. Co., SMA-03=3832. Rockville, MD.

President's New Freedom Commission on Mental Health. (March 5, 2002). Washington, DC: The Executive Office of the President. pp. 22337–22338.

Rural Policy Research Institute. (2016). www.rupri.org.

Wood, R. E. (2008). *Survival of Rural America: Small Victories and Bitter Harvests*. Lawrence: University Press of Kansas.

5 Understanding the Culture of Rural Living

The culture of rural living is an organic conglomerate including families, infants and children, adolescents, women, men, the elderly, indigenous populations, veterans, refugees and undocumented individuals, victims of domestic violence, migrant workers, incarcerated, LGBT, and physical and intellectual disabled and homeless people. Each of these components of rural culture is explored. Weapons ownership is also discussed. Poverty is persistent in rural areas and many cannot find their way out of it, causing it to be intergenerational. Case studies are included.

Although many rural areas appear to have a monoculture, many differences do exist. Some things to consider are differences in social class, education level, religion, race, country versus town residents, farmers versus ranchers, people who live in the floodplain and those who live on high ground. In my own area there are pockets, some not so small, of people who identify as German, Scottish, Irish, Mexican, Jewish, Latino, African American, and Native American. Several ethnic groups have many subgroups, each of which has a different culture, traditions, language, and ancestry. For example, American Indians and Alaska Natives have over 500 tribes, and Asian Americans and Pacific Islanders can be from over 40 subgroups that speak any of over 100 dialects. Rural culture also differs from urban culture with larger numbers of people engaged in seasonal employment, whether they run a farm or a ranch, a ski slope, or a golf course. The rest of the year's income often arrives in the form of unemployment checks.

Many are the dangers inherent in rural life, particularly in farming. These are internalized by the culture and manifest themselves in various ways. They include disproportionately higher rates of mortality from motor vehicle crashes and gun-related incidents, and higher rates of chronic disease and infant mortality. Farming is one of the most dangerous occupations in the world. Farmers have to contend with machine accidents, mad cow and other diseases, anthrax, pesticide exposure, avian flu, and the risk of injury from farm animals.

Most urbanites, many of whom have never been to the country, believe rural culture to be as it appears on stereotypical television shows and movies. Rural characters on shows such as *Ma and Pa Kettle* and *The Beverly Hillbillies* are portrayed as uncultured people who are gullible and tend to fix conflicts through confrontation rather than rational interactions. The result is that what most of us know about rural life is often based on erroneous stereotypes. The *American Gothic* image of rural people as fiercely independent, self-reliant, unsophisticated, and sometimes even ignorant is hard to erase from our collective psyche, although it has some truth to it. Popular television shows such as *The Waltons, Mayberry RFD,* and *Little House on the Prairie* portray rural life more realistically for the times they are meant to portray yet through a romantic haze. *Green Acres* is a sitcom from the 1960s in which a wealthy urban couple played by Eddie Albert and Eva Gabor gives up their New York City penthouse to buy a farm. It features a cast of country characters based on outdated stereotypes juxtaposed onto the glossy urbanites. Josephine the plumber, the jabbering extension agent Hank Kimball, the local huckster Mr. Haney, and Arnold the Pig were among these earthy characters that helped make the show the huge success that it was.

Families

Focusing on the family unit strengthens both the family and the individuals within that family. It also educates parents on ways to parent better. Families these days are found in mostly non-traditional forms. Many are the single-parent households, but the form of family growing exponentially is the grandparents who are raising their grandchildren without the involvement of their children, the parents of those children. If it weren't for these grandparents stepping up to raise their grandchildren, most of these kids would be in foster care. This form of family is referred to as kinship care.

The National Association on Mental Illness (NAMI) offers a program called Family-to-Family. It is a free 12-week course for families, partners, and friends of individuals with serious mental illness, and is taught by more than 3,500 specially trained NAMI family members and caregivers of individuals living with mental illness. The course dwells on the emotional responses families have to the trauma of mental illness; many family members describe their experience in the program as life changing, and I have observed this firsthand. NAMI also offers a Family Support Group Program, also free, which is a monthly meeting of caregivers of individuals with a mental illness where family members can talk frankly about their challenges and help one another through their learned wisdom. NAMI offers many other programs. Check to see which are available on www.nami.org.

Men

Rural men experience more health risk factors, poorer health, and higher death rates than rural women. Of particular concern is their elevated rate of suicide. It is well established that men are four times as likely to commit suicide as women, and this has been found both in the United States and abroad.

Factors that contribute to the high suicide rates of rural men are greater access to guns and other weapons, greater difficulty accessing health and mental health services, greater levels of denial and reluctance in seeking help, and greater difficulty making a living and accessing higher education. According to Dougherty, farm men are more exposed to financial and job-related stress, but less prone to marriage conflict than non-farmers.

International research repeatedly shows that rural men living in different countries have many common characteristics. Among these are a high value on self-reliance, stubbornness, and self-isolation during difficult times. Being diagnosed with a mental illness is perceived as a sign of weakness. This often results in a sustained degree of denial until the problem becomes a crisis. Visiting any kind of health care provider is often a last resort. In addition, rural men generally engage in a higher degree of risky behaviors, including more dangerous levels of drinking alcohol and substance abuse, overworking their bodies or being too sedentary, smoking, and ignoring signs of disease. When a man does decide to seek help from a mental health practitioner, their physician is usually the first stop. Waiting lists, limited treatment options, and traveling long distances can discourage a man who has finally reached out for help to the point that he may not follow through at all. Some mental health professionals believe that many rural men are having difficulty adjusting to the changing gender roles of the past few decades, including the increased numbers of women who are household breadwinners, the increased divorce rate, or the shame of losing the family farm.

Community education about mental health and substance abuse issues will help all people recognize symptomology as well as reduce stigma in seeking help. It will also empower people to heal and recover. In addition to engaging in mental health services, some community-based approaches to helping rural men with mental health issues are men's groups, and involvement with civic, religious, or social organizations, which are outside the home and inadvertently help people feel needed, supported, and wanted. These can be bowling or darts teams, book discussion groups, sports leagues, or hobby groups. Unfortunately, men's groups are rare, but can easily be low cost supplements to reduce isolation, decrease risky behaviors such as substance abuse, and empower men to take care of their mental and physical health needs.

Women

Although over 28 million women of reproductive age live in rural American counties, 43% of rural counties in the United States had no hospital-based obstetric services in 2002, and research shows the number of rural hospitals providing obstetric care and birth options is decreasing. This means more travel for pregnant women for both prenatal care and giving birth. Pre- and post-partum depression in rural women is a topic that needs further research because rural women are often geographically distanced from others with whom they can socialize.

Depression rates for women in rural areas are equal to or higher than those in urban areas, and depressed individuals are nine times more likely to be hospitalized in rural areas as in urban settings. They are twice as likely as men to suffer from major depression, anxiety, and obsessive-compulsive disorder. These types of mental illness often lead to addictive behaviors and social choices contributing to the staggering cost of mental health treatment in the United States. Of all mental illnesses, eating disorders are the number one cause of mortality for women. Much more research is needed in the area of rural women's mental health.

Many women living in rural areas are disproportionately poor, which further limits their already limited resources. Many live in isolated areas with limited opportunities for work, social encounters, and health care. At the same time, they are faced with increased childcare and household/farm responsibilities, and they are more likely to buy into traditional gender roles that can bar them from educational and work opportunities while often living in chauvinistic roles.

Infants and Children

Infant mental health is an area that is rapidly growing in acceptance, with post-graduate certificates now available in infant and child mental health (ages 0–5). Too many community-based mental health centers do not see children under 5. It has been empirically proven that early childhood mental health consultation is an effective strategy for supporting young children's social and emotional development and addressing challenging behaviors in early care and education settings. As a result, more and more states and communities are investing in these programs. They involve a professional consultation with a mental health professional who works collaboratively with early care and education staff in programs such as Head Start and others, and also collaborates with families in order to improve their ability to prevent, screen for, and respond to mental issues among the young children in their care. This approach, in contrast to direct therapeutic services, offers an indirect approach to reducing problem behaviors in young children and helps promote positive social and emotional development.

Providing mental health services to young, preschool children brings up a great deal of controversy. According to the National Advisory Committee on Rural Health and Human Services, 81% of counties with persistent child poverty are non-metropolitan. I've met many practitioners who will not treat children under the age of 5, and some won't even treat children under the age of 12. It has been empirically proven over and over that the earlier the intervention after adverse childhood experiences (ACEs), the more the child's neuropsychological development will catch up to the appropriate developmental level, rather than leaving them lagging behind and in emotional pain.

Exposure to a wide variety of other ACEs during childhood, including physical, emotional, and sexual abuse and neglect, has a strong relationship to a host of health problems over the course of a lifetime, and is recognized as a form of trauma. Congress should amend the Head Start Act to promote trauma-informed practices, age-appropriate, positive behavioral intervention and support services for young children who have experienced trauma, complex trauma, or toxic stress, and improved coordination between Head Start agencies and other programs that serve very young children. Additional funding for mental health consultations is sorely needed.

In my county, the psychiatrist works part time and does not see children younger than 12 years of age. There are also several psychiatric nurse practitioners who could prescribe medication to children, but they are required to work under and follow the preferences of their supervising psychiatrist. The Department of Education should integrate mental health screening, services, and support requirements into Early Start and Head Start to identify and address behavioral health problems early and appropriately.

The Federal Office of Rural Health Policy reports that a research project from the Centers for Disease Control and Prevention looked at available data reported by parents of children between the ages of 2 and 8 throughout the United States and concluded that in rural areas, one in six children was diagnosed with mental, behavioral, and developmental disorders. At 18.6%, the acknowledgement of these diagnoses in rural children was higher than urban children at 15.2%. Factors that were common for families in rural communities include experiencing financial difficulties in which it is hard to pay for food and housing basics, living in neighborhoods with limited amenities such as the lack of sidewalks, community centers, and libraries, and the lack of medical providers of all kinds. In conclusion, they listed three main recommendations, which would be appropriate in both urban and rural settings. They are:

- Collaborations among health care providers, school-based services, and community and state agencies can improve access behavioral health while lowering cost and improving quality.
- School-based services and telemedicine options have both been shown to increase access to behavioral health while reducing stigma and transportation barriers.
- Support for parents that is early and continuous can promote healthy environments for learning experiences within the home.

Since the beginning of the current century, experts have had to address the astronomic rise in the number of children diagnosed and treated for psychological disturbances such as attention deficit hyperactivity disorder (ADHD), autism, mood disorders, and learning disabilities. For example, the number of children diagnosed with autism has grown from 1 in 10,000 in the 1970s to 1 in 63 children and 1 in 42 boys. Pop psychology provides us with generally two viewpoints. The first is that these disturbances are caused by genetically influenced chemical balances in the brain. Magic wand cures are provided in the form of pills to correct these imbalances. Public education and improved diagnostics explain part of the rise of these disorders.

The second explanation is that children, by definition, are inattentive and moody and they need to run and play. In *Childhood Lost*, Sharna Olfman writes that neither of these perspectives tells the whole story. She proposes that some children *are* diagnosed unnecessarily because their behavior is troublesome to adults. Our society has created some unhealthy trends that undermine children's psychological health, such as developmentally insensitive school systems, the disappearance of creative play in early childhood, and screen technologies that remove them from essential developmental tasks, such as physical activity, and immerse them in violent and sexualized worlds. At the same time, many children are struggling with very real symptoms ranging from impulsivity and learning challenges to panic and rage. So we ask whether solutions lie in fixing their biology or fixing their environments. In *The Science and Pseudoscience of Children's Mental Health*, she strongly suggests that we are asking the wrong question. Nature versus nurture is an outdated dichotomy that has been replaced in serious scientific circles by the science of epigenetics. In short, epigenetics involves understanding that environments, whether they be cellular or social, can activate or silence genes, which has a profound effect on brain development.

According to neurobiologist Richard Francis, as quoted in *The Science and Pseudoscience of Children's Mental Health*, recognizing the role of environment in regulating gene behavior unleashes enormous potential for understanding children's mental health and developing interventions ranging from diet to relationships, which in turn alter gene expression. The standardized view, which focuses on identifying an ADHD gene or gene sequence with an intention treatment at the gene level, with no consideration of the role of environment, is shortsighted and fundamentally flawed. The science of epigenetics has taught us that when we look at a child's environment holistically, by allowing them to limit their time spent outdoors in nature in favor of spending hours sitting in front of screens; feeding them food that is processed and tainted with insecticides rather than fresh foods; living with polluted air, soil, and water that is saturated with tens of thousands of man-made chemical toxins, a thousand of which have been targeted as neuro or brain toxins, that these environments powerfully impact gene expression, and brain development. It stands to reason.

Rural Matters: Alone on a Hilltop

The house stands alone, atop a hill on a dirt road. It is 3 miles uphill from the village. The boards outside the house are weathered, like dry scaly skin. An assortment of large plastic playthings peppers the front lawn, strewn as if the wind arranged them. Wind blows the tall, yellowed grass surrounding the outskirts of the house. The blades look bleak against the deep gray sky. Intermittent flocks of geese fly through, trying to escape this forsaken place.

A dim light shines from inside the front window. Dusk falls quickly, the sounds from town muffled. A pale light by the front door slivers the darkness. When night falls here, it falls with a thud. Blackness, solid as pavement, isolates these inhabitants.

Inside, a mother and her son are in the kitchen. Supper is on the table. The boy is 3 years old; the mother is in her late thirties. Supper is macaroni and cheese from a box. The kitchen is sparse, lacking in the way of conveniences. Both mother and son are wearing sweaters to keep warm and conserve wood. The wood stove is a bottomless pit at this time of year, and who knows when the man of the house will return to cut more firewood.

This is where their life happens—the only home the boy has known. His mother is one of a handful of people he has met in his life. Mom knows how to drive, but has no car. Dad has gone way south to work, 12 hours' drive to where he has steady work. He comes home when he can, about every three or four weeks. Even so, he is only able to stay for a few days, say two or three, before he must return. He could have found work in West Virginia in the coal mines, but being on the road crew in South Carolina is safer and easier work, and besides, it pays better. It's double the distance, but for safety's sake they agreed on it.

She met him in her early thirties after a bad marriage left her feeling defeated. A girlfriend she waited on tables with introduced them, and they liked each other right away. Back then he worked in the Pennsylvania coal slag heaps. That was only a 2-hour ride. They moved in together before long, into his little house on the hill, and it wasn't long before she was pregnant. The boy was born in the spring, making it easy to get out for walks and rides. It was a happy time for the young family, with no thought of the future. The present was all there was.

Slowly the leaves turned color, the temperature dropped, and the sky turned what seemed a permanent gray. It wasn't until the lavender asters appeared that the family gave any thought to what life on their little hill would be like through the winter. Once the baby arrived, they agreed he would take a job farther away on the road crews in order to get higher wages. She cherished the time she had to be home with their only child, and besides, her intellect and skills were limited. She gave motherhood her all.

The first snowflakes fell midweek while her man was down south. Along with it were millions of others forming mounds of white on their hill outside of town, and it was on that hill the boy and his mother stayed through most of the winter. When the man was home, he saw that they were stocked up with enough food and wood, and there was very little else they needed. Every once in a while, her girlfriend would see if she could make it up the hill and take them into town for whatever they needed.

When the boy turned 3, the man said he thought he should start school. He heard about a program for preschoolers in which a bus would pick the child up and then deliver him back home again. As hard as it was to separate herself from the boy, she listened to his reasoning. She agreed to send him to school, which was 5 days a week during the school year. When the boy got to school, the staff found it very difficult to understand his speech. They realized he had few social skills and none of the academic preparation most parents do with their preschoolers in the areas of alphabet, number and color recognition, naming animals, and singing songs. He knew little of any of that. When he tried to make himself heard, no one understood his words. He played by himself while his classmates were beginning to move from parallel play to real interacting. He was lost. And, he missed his mother. Sometimes for weeks and weeks she was the only person he saw. She was his alpha and his omega, and almost everything in between.

Adolescents

Rural adolescents tend to drink more alcohol and have higher rates of risky sexual behavior than their urban counterparts. Youth who abuse alcohol and illegal substances such as methamphetamines and inhalants are now more prevalent in rural areas (14%) than urban areas (10%). As a result of substance abuse, rural youth are also more likely than urban youth to engage in dangerous behavior such as binge drinking, heavy drinking, and driving under the influence. They are two times more likely to be sexually active and to become sexually active at a younger age (Health Resources and Services Administration, HRSA). A recent report by the Centers for Disease Control (CDC) examined current alcohol use and binge drinking among high school students in the United States between the years of 1991 and 2015. Their results revealed that approximately one in three high school students drank alcohol during the past 30 days, and one in six was a binge drinker.

In 2017, a new measurement category was unveiled by the Federal Office of Rural Health Policy. Called "disconnected youth," it studied young adults aged 16–24 who are not in school and also not working. The findings suggest that these youths are more prevalent in rural areas than urban. The agency also reports that premature deaths increased the most among those between the ages of 15 and 44. Drug overdose was the single leading cause of premature death by injury in 2015, but for those aged 15–24, more deaths due to motor vehicle crashes and firearm fatalities also played a role in the accelerated rise. A recent study by the Center for Rural Entrepreneurship found that half of the young people from rural communities said that they would love to settle down in their hometowns if career opportunities awaited them. The irony for our young adults is that too many of them are economically forced out of metropolitan areas to settle in less expensive areas, and many seek a less hectic lifestyle more in tune with nature and open space. Conversely, many rural young adults are forced to leave their rural homes in order to make an adequate living. Many find the city expenses and lifestyle unmanageable and return for the wrong reasons. It's hard for them to thrive either way, too often. And those of us who have raised our children in small rural communities want the opportunity of having our children settle here and raise their own families close by.

Given the statistics for alcohol and drug abuse among rural youth, screenings and prevention programs need to be widespread and easily accessible with reduced stigma, with the focus on middle and high schoolers. For those rural adolescents who engage in substance abuse, research shows that they have a higher chance of achieving higher remission rates when in treatment for a year. There was also evidence that rural youth require more aftercare compared to urban youth, which presents a greater need not only for substance abuse treatments but also follow-up methods of intervention.

Suicide among rural adolescents has been shown to be higher than the rate for their urban counterparts—some studies showing a 15% increase. According to Smalley et al. in *Rural Mental Health*, many factors have been identified as driving these disparities in suicide rates, including access to lethal means, geographic and social isolation, and mental health stigma. These factors are even more striking among adolescents, sometimes demonstrated to be 15 times higher among rural adolescents when compared to urban.

The Elderly

Overall, rural areas have a disproportionate number of elderly citizens. According to the National Advisory Committee on Rural Health and Human Services, approximately 7.5 million of the 50 million people living in rural America in 2005 were over age 65. They report that although the difference in percentage of the elderly between rural and urban areas is only 12% versus 9%, the rural elderly population is growing at a faster rate. Rural residents make up approximately 25% of the Medicare population, and 30% of Medicare beneficiaries who also qualify for Medicaid live in rural America. Many of these people are not offered a prescription drug coverage plan. Given the scant infrastructure of rural health care, this presents a significant challenge.

The elderly have complex mental health needs, sometimes including dementia, feelings of hopelessness due to aging, and end of life issues. Growing old involves so many losses. Many elderly people have lost friends and relatives, their children may live far from them, and they often experience a loss of health. Their roles have shifted to being retired, possibly widowed, and our society tends to devalue them. They are forced to live on fixed incomes. Many older adults have relinquished their driver's licenses, making the distance needed to travel for services more difficult to bridge. Increased outreach by local offices for aging and senior citizens is needed to alleviate the isolation many elderly rural residents feel due to geographic distances, including senior meal sites, social gathering places, bus transportation to events and appointments, and educational outreach programs to educate the public about issues their elderly friends and neighbors face. Programming need not be costly. Adopt-a-grandparent programs, in which children visit senior residences, perhaps have a snack, or do an art or music project together, don't cost anything.

A higher percentage of rural elderly live below the federal poverty level compared to the urban elderly. Depending on the source, the elderly are often referred to as having the highest suicide rate in our country.

For those who can no longer live independently, there is a severe shortage of assisted-living and skilled nursing facilities, and for those that do exist, a severe shortage of qualified staff. In order to age in place, which most of us would prefer to do, we need many more qualified nurses, occupational, physical, and mental health therapists to be itinerant. For that to happen, there need to be better salaries, more vacation time, and other perks to attract them to serve rural areas.

Indigenous Populations: American Indians and Alaska Natives

American Indians and Alaska Natives occupy a special place in the history and folklore of America. Their very existence is a testament to their collective and individual spirit and culture. According to the 2000 census, about 4.1 million American Indians and Alaska Natives live in our country, representing less than 1.5% of the population. They are unique citizens in that they are members of federally recognized sovereign nations that exist within another country.

They were victims of the unintentional spread of infectious disease as European white folks landed on our shores in the 1600s. The immune systems of the indigenous population were unable to fight off the diseases brought unknowingly by European settlers. Successive history shows them enduring violent attacks and being chased off their land by white settlers. All this collective trauma has an ongoing effect on the trust these populations have in our government and sets the stage for understanding their mental health needs.

There are 561 federally recognized tribes speaking over 200 indigenous languages. This often necessitates providing treatment in their native language or at least not in English. Given the shortage of mental health practitioners in rural and frontier areas, this is often impossible. Interestingly enough, many words such as "depressed" and "anxious" don't exist in some of these languages. In addition, other research has shown that certain diagnoses from the DSM, such as major depressive disorder, do not correspond directly to the categories of illness recognized by some American Indians. Therefore, evaluating the need for mental health care among American Indians and Alaska Natives requires extra careful clinical inquiry that correlates to culture.

Although little research has been done on rates of psychiatric disorders among American Indians and Alaska Natives in the United States, one nationally representative study looked at mental health among a large sample of adults (Centers for Disease Control and Prevention, 2011). Overall, American Indians and Alaska Natives reported much higher rates of frequent distress, nearly 13% compared to nearly 9% within the general population. These findings suggest that these indigenous cultures experience greater psychological distress than the overall population. Many culturally based expressions of distress include what these cultures refer to as "heartbreak syndrome" and "ghost sickness." This brings up the question of how to elicit, understand, and incorporate these expressions of anguish into the assessment and treatment process we use in our medical model, which is based on the DSM.

The suicide rate for this ethnic minority group was 1.5 times the national rate. The suicide rate is particularly high among young Native American males aged between 15 and 24. Accounting for 64% of all suicides by American Indians and Alaska Natives, the rate of this group is two to three times higher than the rate for the general US population. It is important to note that violent deaths, which include unintentional injuries, homicide, and suicide, account for 75% of all mortality in the second decade of life for these ethnic groups. It is no coincidence that they are the most impoverished ethnic minority group in America today and are overrepresented among the homeless population. Although they account for less than 1% of America's general population, American Indians and Alaska Natives account for 8% of our country's homeless population. Let there be no doubt: poverty, homelessness, and mental illness are interconnected.

Although little research has been done on the rates of substance abuse in this population, evidence suggests that a substantial proportion suffers from alcoholism, with rates varying greatly from tribe to tribe. Rural Native Americans do not differ from urban Native American populations in rates of alcohol abuse, which are higher than the population at large; however, rural Native Americans tend to have more episodes of binge drinking. Given the higher than average rates of alcohol abuse in the American Indian and Alaska Native population, fetal alcohol syndrome (FAS) is an important cause of mental health needs within these populations. FAS is now recognized as the leading cause of intellectual disability in the United States. FAS is a disorder that continues for a lifetime in a predictable pattern of long-term progression with a collection of maladaptive behaviors including poor judgment, distractibility, difficulty perceiving social cues, and a high need for intervention in order for them to be participating members of society.

American Indian youth drinking rates have been studied more often than adult rates. Research has shown that although about the same proportion of Indian and non-Indian youth in grades 7–12 have tried alcohol, Indian youth who drink appear to drink more heavily than do youth in the general population and experience more negative social consequences from this behavior than their non-Indian peers. Trauma may be responsible for this, as research has also shown that in an investigation of Northern Plains youth between the ages of 8 and 11, 61% of them had been exposed to some kind of traumatic event. Other studies show 82% had been exposed to one traumatic event, and the prevalence of post-traumatic stress disorder (PTSD) was 22%, making it appear as though these populations have greater rates of trauma exposure. Much more research needs to be done on these populations in order to serve their needs satisfactorily. In addition, there are approximately 101 Native Americans and Alaska Native mental health providers of all types available per 100,000 people in these ethnic groups, as compared with over 173 per 100,000 for white segments of the population.

When it comes to accessibility to mental health care, most Alaska Natives and many American Indians live in frontier areas, making transportation a significant issue. As stated previously, there are more caribou than people in Alaska, and over 40% of the population has a pilot's license. Nevertheless, the cost of getting to a mental or physical health appointment by air is exorbitant.

A final point about these indigenous populations is that their cultures have very deep roots many do not wish to give up. Research shows that in many cases American Indians and Alaska natives use alternative therapies at rates that are equal to or greater than the rates for whites. One study found that 63% of

Navajo patients interviewed at a rural clinic had used native healers, and 39% reported using them on a regular basis. For those who were not using a native healer currently, 9 out of 10 would consider using one in the future. And these populations are quick to observe that the public health model that deals with prevention of mental illness is a disease-oriented model of care. Professionals are encouraged by members of these indigenous groups to move beyond these models and the separation of mind, body, and spirit and consider individual as well as collective strengths in the promotion of mental health.

Veterans—Visible and Invisible Injuries

According to the U.S. Defense Department, there are more than 22 million veterans in the United States. Of them, 5.3 million live in rural areas. For decades, we've known that rural communities turn over more of their young people to the military than urban areas, and by extension, during wartime, experience more casualties and losses. With our country still fighting the longest war in the history of our nation, it is more important than ever to ensure that all veterans receive as much physical and mental health care as they need. Research indicates that veterans are more likely to seek treatment through Veterans Administration (VA) facilities than through non-VA mental health services. And yet the vast majority of those who are able to utilize VA services have lower levels of usage than the general population. In recent years there have been huge issues in VA services, long waiting periods for services in some cases. Many rural residents have to travel hours in order to access VA services.

On average, there are 22 suicides of American active duty military and veterans every day. Dougherty found that among soldiers and veterans with PTSD and a history of torture, a correlation was found between the torture methods that the victim had been exposed to and the suicide method used in ideation or attempts. Dougherty wrote that blunt force applied to the head and body was associated with jumping from a height or in front of trains, water torture was equated with drowning, and sharp force torture with methods involving self-inflicted stabbing or cutting. It is probable that those who were exposed to more severe circumstances such as losing a friend in battle or being taken prisoner will be more at risk. As we know, individual levels of resilience are likely to vary from person to person for a variety of reasons. More than 43% of veterans who committed suicide did not seek help from military treatment facilities in the month prior to their deaths. Combat or survivor's guilt has been shown in some studies to be a strong predictor of suicidal thoughts and attempts.

What can we offer these brave men and women in uniform when some return from combat to rural areas with PTSD and so few mental health resources? Once back on home soil, many of the men and women in our armed forces assist with natural disasters, support the active military in various ways, or become members of the National Guard and Reserve, first responders, firefighters, Civil Air Patrol, and other highly trained functions. The main function of crisis counseling with this vulnerable population should be to protect them from further harm while providing a safe, non-judgmental relationship in which they can learn to manage their emotions and begin the long healing process. The therapeutic relationship should help them slowly return to a state of homeostasis, albeit a post-traumatic version. We need to give these veterans back the power to serve their own lives. Their injuries are often invisible from the outside, while bleeding on the inside.

PTSD, with its list of debilitating symptoms, is now being recognized and diagnosed more frequently than in prior wars, including the Vietnam War. It has become the trademark of the wars in Iraq and Afghanistan. According to Hansley (in Dougherty and Mitchell, 2013),

> rural regions of the Midwest and other areas of the United States are ill prepared to address the emerging crisis posited to become multigenerational. We must endeavor to understand the foundations of PTSD rather than assigning contrite criteria to diagnose and eradicate externalized symptomology rather than addressing the insidious causal etiology.
>
> (xi)

PTSD is diagnosed by determining the presence of a set of symptoms, which include depression, rage, anxiety, survivor's guilt, intrusive thoughts, isolation, and avoidance of feelings. The DSM-5 lists a specific list of symptoms and their duration for qualification. When one member of a close family is traumatized, the rest of the family members are at risk of vicarious or secondary traumatization, as are mental health workers. When untreated and unresolved, it becomes chronic and sometimes intergenerational. PTSD often leads to job instability, poverty, obsessive-compulsive disorder, sleep disorders, divorce, social phobias, somatization disorder, and child and/or spousal abuse or other kind of physical aggression. It is also associated with increased methods of working with such families can include psychoeducational, behavioral, psychodynamic, systematic, and even spiritual methodologies.

If the VA does not have enough mental health practitioners on staff, they need to either increase their staff or hire outside consultants to keep up with the high needs our veterans have.

Refugees and Undocumented Immigrants

The Trump administration thrust refugees and illegal immigrants to the forefront to become the top hot-button issue of the 2016 presidential campaign and throughout all of 2017. Pockets of many nationalities from all over the globe can be found in America's rural areas. Refugees are often seeking safety and a job for themselves and their families. Illegal immigrants are often transient because of their strong connection to agriculture and harvesting. If deported, many would be leaving behind children who were born in this country. If both parents are deported and no other relatives can be found nearby, those children will likely enter the foster care system at the expense of the American taxpayer with little regard for their mental health and well-being.

Many in each of these groups have PTSD and attachment issues from the separation of their family members. Many have experienced abuse or torture, and many suffer from social adjustment issues related to their experiences. Language and cultural barriers sometimes stand in the way of these populations getting treatment. Many are the cultural differences in how emotional issues are viewed. For example, there are traditional Mexican folk illnesses such as *susto*, a condition that can include symptoms such as sleep disturbance, gastrointestinal issues, depression, and a general feeling of listlessness brought about by a sudden shock. *Nervios* is a group of symptoms that may include anxiety, agitation, depression, and nervousness. If they do seek treatment, mental health professionals must understand the issues. There have been few, if any, studies on these populations in rural areas, making it critical for more research to be done. All this adds up to the importance of mental health professionals in rural areas having increased knowledge and training in working with refugees, illegal immigrants, and trauma survivors—in short, being culturally competent.

Migrant Workers

Migrant workers and their families have a high degree of mental health needs. By definition they are migratory, often traveling as families with children who learn not to become too attached to people, places, or situations. The National Advisory Council on Migrant Health (NACMH) was founded in 1975 to advise, consult, and make recommendations to the Secretary of Health and Human Services and the HRSA administrator concerning everything that has to do with operating migrant health centers. This includes but is not limited to the organization, selection, and funding of the migrant health centers. Frequent mobility, long working days, low wages, limited or no benefits, language and cultural differences, separation from loved ones, and discrimination or harassment on the job can all be strong factors contributing to poor states.

Fatalism is a predominant belief among Latino culture. It is the idea that problems with one's health or emotions are beyond an individual's control. Research has shown that Latinos with depression are less likely to find antidepressants an acceptable form of treatment and are less likely to engage in therapy. Their preferred methods of alleviating depression include alcohol abuse and illicit drugs such as crack cocaine, heroin, opioids, and others. One study determined that the frequency of substance abuse was not necessarily tied to ethnicity but rather related to the type of crop work a person works on, because some crops are more labor-intensive than others, making them more physically demanding and stressful. In addition, those with depressive symptoms, which often cause daytime sleepiness, are especially dangerous as these workers often require the use of heavy machinery, tools, toxic pesticides, and heavy lifting. A 2008 national study found that 60% of whites with depression received treatment as opposed to only 36% of Latinos. Research also shows that Latinos are discouraged from seeking mental health treatment due to the cultural insensitivity, stereotyping, and unacknowledged racism they have experienced with professionals.

Victims of Domestic Violence (DV)

According to the National Advisory Committee on Rural Health and Human Services, Domestic violence is a serious mental and physical health issue that affects one in three women in the United States and an unknown number of men and children. Of these women, over one-third have experienced more than one of these behaviors from an intimate partner, and most people who experience domestic violence first experience it before they are 25 years old. The abuse can be verbal or physical, and can range from rape and physical assault to stalking and emotional manipulation. The committee reports that research shows that between 30% and 60% of the families where domestic violence or the maltreatment of children is identified, it is likely that both forms of abuse exist. Women who have experienced domestic violence in rural areas are more likely to be murdered by a partner than those living in cities.

One study found that 22.9% of women in small rural areas reported being victims of domestic violence compared to 15.5% of women in urban areas. The study also found that women living in rural communities reported significantly higher severity of physical abuse than women living in urban areas. Interestingly enough, in 2006, the Centers for Disease Control (CDC) discontinued its policy of allowing researchers to access restricted information in the Behavioral Risk Factor Surveillance System (BRFSS) datasets from respondents in counties with 10,000 or fewer residents that is suppressed in the publicly available datasets. As a result of this change, the BRFSS data could no longer be used to analyze rural domestic violence. Several smaller studies support the findings that the rates of domestic violence are equally as high or higher in rural areas than those in urban communities.

Domestic violence often leads to debilitating and often permanent physical and mental damage. Many states have DV prevention laws that mandate that counties provide domestic violence services.

Those who are victims of the abuse are more likely to experience extreme fear, concern for their safety as well as the safety of their children, physical injury and the need for medical treatment, a need for safe housing should they decide to leave their situation, and missed time at work, which is particularly difficult if the victim is an hourly employee with no sick time.

Many are the shared characteristics of the batterers as well as their victims. And many are the diagnoses victims may have as a result. They include but are not limited to PTSD, major depressive disorder, dissociative symptoms or full blown dissociative disorder, acute stress disorder, and other kinds of anxiety and depression disorders. Victims of domestic violence show an increased risk for asthma, irritable bowel syndrome, and diabetes, as well as poor mental health. Battered women who seek help in a rural area face the possibility that law enforcement officials, judges, members of social services, and physicians may have a personal relationship with either the victim or her abuser.

Also, patriarchal attitudes in certain cultures pose challenges for providing community resources in rural areas. Another study of rural primary care physicians noted that 32% of rural primary care physicians perceived that cultural expectations common to rural communities tend to establish domestic violence as normal behavior, with beliefs that a woman is subservient to a man accepted as the norm. Lack of cell phone service, lack of a permanent address if the victim leaves the perpetrator, lack of good quality affordable housing, and shelters that are filled to capacity are all barriers to a victim of domestic violence changing his or her life. One person in my community pointed out that if you live miles up in a hollow and don't have a landline telephone, a cell phone isn't going to work up there, and if you don't have a car, don't read or write very well, and have young children at home, how are you going to get help?

According to the Committee on Rural Health and Human Services, in a qualitative study in Kentucky where both rural and urban women who had applied for orders of protection were asked about coping strategies, more urban women sought talking to a friend or talking to family, while rural women were more likely to be dealing with their experiences alone. Rural women were more likely to report containing their feelings and trying to ignore the abuse than urban women, who were more likely to suggest they were optimistic about their future and were empowered to take steps to change their situation. I know from my own experiences that when orders of protection are in place in small towns, they can be difficult to enforce because of the increased chances of running into someone unexpectedly because there are not a lot of alternatives to shopping, schools, doctors, and so forth. I have seen parents with restraining orders against them prohibited from stepping on school property. As a result, they have to pick their children up a block away, miss plays, concerts, and sporting events because these events take place on school grounds.

In 40%–75% of families where DV occurs, children are experiencing physical abuse at the same time and are at greater risk of being sexually abused, according to the New York State Coalition Against Domestic Violence. Children who experience or witness DV may develop sleep disorders, regression, extreme fear, low self-esteem, withdrawal, a disruptive sense of autonomy, feelings of utter helplessness, disruptions in the ability to distinguish between reality and fantasy or outright dissociation, increased aggressive behavior, uncontrolled anger or tantrums, hypervigilance, and more. So is a young child who can't sit still in a classroom showing signs of ADHD or showing hyperarousal symptoms from trauma exposure?

On a more positive note, the New York State Coalition Against Domestic Violence found that 40% or more children exposed to domestic violence are resilient, meaning that they are doing at least as well as children who were not exposed to DV. They also found that 37%–40% of children who witnessed or personally experienced abuse fared as well or better than children who did not experience DV.

From a rehabilitative point of view, there is a severe scarcity of programs for men that address battering. We need to set up such programs in as many rural areas as possible in order to break the cycle. Much of this behavior is intergenerational, and unless there are viable treatment programs that can help these men understand and have support in changing their behavior, the cycle will continue.

In conclusion, it is critical that we provide services to victims of domestic violence that is empowering, safe, trauma informed, and administered by professionals who understand the nature and dynamics of DV.

Incarcerated Populations and Sex Offenders

Patrick Kennedy says of decarceration that every county in the United States should be implementing a system whereby they divert individuals with serious mental illness or co-occurring substance use disorders into community-based treatment and support services instead of putting them in jail. And for those already incarcerated with mental illnesses, states should adopt a version of the Mentally Ill Offender Community Transition Program from Washington State, a collaboration between the Department of Corrections and the Department of Mental Health that made a large impact on recidivism rates.

The ever-increasing number of individuals with mental illness who are being incarcerated in the nation's over 3,600 county and local jails has reached crisis levels, according to Ron Manderscheid, director of the National Association of County Behavioral Health and Developmental Disability Directors (NACBHDD). Each year, two million adults with serious mental illnesses, many with co-occurring substance use problems, are routed to jails both before and after sentencing for generally minor infractions. Note that this does not include other millions with behavioral disorders who are housed in state or federal prisons, many with non-violent drug offenses. As a result, the nation's jails have become de facto behavioral health facilities, in which millions of people with treatable mental or substance use disorders are being housed, often with limited treatment and no plans for post-release, community-based care. Little thought is given to actual recovery in the proper sense of the word. Once incarcerated, people with mental illnesses tend to stay longer in jail and are at higher risk of recidivism than individuals without these illnesses. It costs jails two to three times the amount to house people with mental illness than those without. Allowing these individuals to remain in jail or cycle through the criminal system time and time again does nothing to improve their health, continuity of care, or recovery. It also affects public safety and strains local budgets.

The NACBHDD led an unprecedented collaboration with judicial and criminal justice agencies in what might be called a decarceration movement. The result of the collaboration is called *The Stepping Up Initiative*, which is designed to generate action in communities across the country toward the common goal of reducing the number of people with mental illness who are crowding our jails and prisons. Many of these initiatives focus on reforming sentencing guidelines to reduce the reincarceration rate for non-violent drug and parole offenses. The program includes resources designed to help counties develop an action plan that makes better use of budgets, and promotes appropriate alternatives to incarceration for those with behavioral disorders, including the growing numbers of veterans with PTSD and other war-related disorders.

More than 2.7 million children in the United States have an incarcerated parent. Between 1991 and 2007, the number of children with a father in prison grew by 77%, while the number of children with an incarcerated mother grew by 131%. Those numbers continue to explode as the current drug epidemic worsens. For people who become impoverished because of mental illness, if they reach a point where they may pose a danger to themselves or others, they often end up incarcerated, making our prisons treatment centers of last resort. Thus, our jails are overflowing with mentally ill inmates who don't get the mental health treatment they so desperately need.

Parental incarceration wreaks havoc with a child's life in terms of emotions, especially shame and guilt, economics, social and living arrangements, and often intellect, because we know that prolonged stress changes brain chemistry and strong emotions can affect concentration and mood. Separation from a parent due to incarceration can be as traumatic as death or any other kind of separation for children, especially because of the stigma and lack of social support and compassion. Children's reactions to incarceration differ depending on many factors, including the quality of the relationship between the parent and child, the age of the child at the time of separation, and whether or not contact is maintained. All children of incarcerated parents experience the stigma of having a parent imprisoned, and the hopefully temporary loss of the parent they would like to have in their daily lives. Much more research is needed to determine the scope of the ways parental incarceration affects children. Some of what the current research already tells us is that parental incarceration is what the Centers for Disease Control and Prevention (CDC) recognize as an adverse childhood experience. We know that multiple adverse experiences significantly increase the likelihood of long-term negative mental health and health outcomes, and we know that stigma damages self-esteem, causes attachment issues, and may distort a child's sense of trust leading to anger and aggressive behavior. We also know that children of incarcerated parents may be twice as likely as the general population of children to develop mental health problems, higher rates of major depression, and attention disorders.

Bringing Home the Bacon . . . or Not: The Persistence of Poverty

Nearly 85% of persistent poverty counties in the United States are in rural areas, and in many of these areas the high rates of poverty have lasted for generations. Over 6.2 million rural Americans are still living in poverty, and that number includes 1.5 million children. According to Rosalynn Carter in *Within Our Reach*, rural communities still have poverty rates almost 25% higher than urban counties and account for almost 90% of all the "persistent poverty" counties as defined by the USDA, as counties that have experienced poverty rates above 20% for the past 30 years.

Michael Harrington says about poverty in America that, for the economist John Kenneth Galbraith, there are two main components of poverty: case poverty and insular poverty. Case poverty is the plight of those who suffer from some physical or mental disability that is personal and individual and leaves them functioning poorly or not at all. Insular poverty exists in areas like the Appalachians or the West Virginia coal fields, where an entire section of the country becomes perpetually poor. The most familiar form of denial is the view that the poor are that way because they are afraid of work, they spend their money on the wrong things, and prefer to live on the social programs funded by the taxpayers. Harrington wrote that there are two important ways of looking at this phenomenon. The poor are either caught in a vicious circle, or they live in a culture of poverty. Here is one of the most familiar forms of the vicious circle of poverty. Picture a downward spiral. The poor in general have poor diets—have you ever noticed how expensive it is to eat healthy? They tend to get sick more than others in society and often do not have access to adequate medical care. When they become sick, they tend to be sick longer than any other group in our society. Because they are sick more often and longer than anyone else, they lose wages and work, and find it difficult to hold a steady job. And because of this, they cannot pay for good housing, a nutritious diet, or doctors. At any given point, particularly when there is a major illness, their fate very often is to move to an even lower level and to begin the cycle, round and round, toward even more suffering. This is only one example of the vicious circle of poverty.

Finally, Harrington writes of the farming poor that perhaps the harshest and most bitter poverty in the United States is to be found in the farm fields themselves. The irony is that these men and women form their culture of poverty in the midst of abundance—they often go hungry while working fields that produce more than ever before.

According to a research report by Cornell University in 2010, rural poverty changes as rural demographics change. Current trends affecting poverty include the non-traditional nature of family structures, the "brain drain" and out-migration of educated youth, an increasing percentage of senior citizens, and transient and migrant workers in rural economies. The challenges to combating rural poverty include a disconnect between jobs, transportation, and housing; a lack of access of access to health care of all types; an apparent intergenerational cycle of poverty; stigma and general lack of awareness about mental health that prevents people from obtaining help; and competition between programs for a limited amount of available funding.

For more on poverty in rural America, see Chapter 8.

Weapons Ownership

When it comes to gun ownership and Second Amendment rights, twice as many rural residents own guns as in urban areas, and nearly a third more than in suburban areas. There are many reasons people keep guns in their homes. In rural areas, those reasons expand to include hunting and target shooting. And while it is perfectly legal to own a registered gun, many are not locked, making them accessible to children and adolescents. Slovak (2002) conducted a study examining children's exposure to violence in rural settings. In doing so, she explored exposure to violence as well as the psychological trauma linked with that exposure. The results of Slovak's study show that children in the rural sample were exposed to high amounts of violence as a victim and a witness. More boys than girls reported being exposed to violence, with the exception of girls who reported being touched in a private area. More students in lower grades than in upper grades reported being exposed to violence. Students reported that the place they were most likely to be victims of violence was their home, while school was reported as the most likely place to be victimized or to witness violence. And while most students reported the neighborhood as the least likely place they would be most likely to be a victim of violence, it was the second most likely place to witness violence. Not surprisingly, Slovak found that exposure to violence was responsible for a significant increase in anxiety, anger, dissociation, depression, PTSD, and other symptoms, which is consistent with previous studies and at odds with our national attitude toward rural areas as safe havens from violence.

As for gun violence and rural youth, Slovak compared youth in grades 3–8 as to those who were exposed to gun violence versus those who were not. The comparison variables included anger, anxiety, depression, dissociation, PTSD, total trauma, violent behavior, parental monitoring, and levels of violence at home, at school, and in the community at large. Youth exposed to gun violence displayed higher levels of the symptomology listed above and significantly higher levels of violent behaviors, and had lower levels of parental monitoring.

Slovak then studied the relationship between access to firearms and parental monitoring on rural youth's exposure to gun violence, as well as the effect of gun violence exposure on the mental health of these youths. The results of her study showed that a substantial number were exposed to gun violence and that exposure was significantly related to firearm access and parental monitoring. Gun violence exposure was significantly associated with trauma among youths. I count myself among the mental health workers who have had to

Drug and Alcohol Abuse—see Chapter 13 on Substance Abuse

The LGBTQ Population

Sexual and gender identity has smashed through many barriers throughout the world over the past decades. Aside from the usual terms of lesbian, gay, bisexual, transsexual, and questioning people, we now have terms such as pansexual (those who do not feel limited in sexual choice with regard to biological sex, gender, or gender identity) and gender fluid (those who do not identify themselves as having a fixed gender). The subject becomes more complicated all the time—or maybe it always was complicated, but just wasn't dealt with. There is a definite bias in our cultural thinking that anyone in the LGBTQ population is more readily accepted in an urban area. And in some ways this is true. In other ways, it requires more explanation.

A study done by Megan Paceley of the University of Kansas revealed four areas of need for youths in this population: reduction in isolation, social acceptance and visibility, emotional support and safety, and gender and sexual minority identity development. Community support was overwhelmingly voted the top need. The study quotes participants as stating that support can come in many forms, including simply having businesses post a rainbow flag in their window. Teachers in some schools have posted rainbow flags in the windows of their doors so students will know which faculty and staff members are gay friendly. Emotional support and safety—both physical and emotional—were other huge needs. Participants mentioned the need for LGBTQ-savvy school counselors and safe shelters in case intolerant parents tossed kids out onto the street. These also need to be accepting, as some religious-based shelters will not take in LGBTQ individuals, and some gender-specific shelters will not take in transgendered people.

Legal support would be helpful to many for several reasons. Some, as in the case of transgendered people, may need a legal change of name. Others may need legal assistance in order to know how to navigate the new rules and laws surrounding public bathroom use. We need more schools and civic organizations to start gay–straight alliance groups for emotional support and companionship. These organizations can also help with learning how to come out to family, for sharing legal and emotional information, and for understanding new terms such as cisgender or pansexual.

A few words on conversion therapy, which became popular in the 1980s and 1990s and which was designed to try to convert individuals who identified as gay and lesbian into becoming straight. Homosexuality, its proponents claimed, is a "curable disorder." To give some perspective to the timeline of conversion therapy, the American Psychiatric Association voted to remove homosexuality from its list of mental health disorders in 1974, just when conversion therapy was taking off in popularity. This type of therapy was found to be so dangerous to participants that President Obama proposed a national ban on it in 2015.

Sometimes referred to as reparative therapy, it was found to drive a majority of participants to depression, anxiety, drug use, or suicide. Initially, the Christian right was the loudest voice in favor of conversion therapy. Because large pockets of the Christian right reside in rural areas, rural community members who identified as homosexual were even more alienated in their own communities than their urban counterparts, and probably more bullied and mistreated. By the beginning of the current decade, the scientific foundation of reparative therapy eroded, every major medical association renounced it, and the movement is dying. According to the *Atlantic*, the death knell sounded in July of 2013 when Alan Chambers, president of Exodus International, America's largest ex-gay Christian ministry, apologized to the LGBT community and shut down his organization. Virtually every major medical and mental health related organization opposes conversion therapy, and some states have made it officially illegal, at least for minors.

As mental health professionals, we have a unique opportunity to be at the forefront of supporting these individuals. In rural areas, we can really forge new paths and ways to support this population. It is our privilege to do so.

A good source of information on this subject is the Gay, Lesbian, and Straight Educational Network (GLSEN). The book *Strengths and Silences: The Experience of LGBT Students in Rural and Small Schools* can be downloaded free of charge from their website at www.glsen.org.

A few statistics on the experience of LGBTQ students in rural areas describes their experience well:

- Nearly all LGBTQ students in rural areas have heard homophobic, racist, sexist, and negative gender expression–based remarks, and more frequently than urban and suburban students.
- Ninety-seven percent of rural LGBT students heard words such as "gay" used derogatorily at school.
- Rural students were more likely than suburban or urban students to hear most types of biased language. More than 25% of students heard staff make homophobic or negative remarks about gender.
- At least 81% of rural LGBTQ students had felt unsafe at school during the past year because of a personal characteristic. Sexual orientation and gender expression were the most common reasons rural students said they felt unsafe.
- Students in the South and Midwest were more likely to feel unsafe than rural students in the West and Northeast.
- Nearly 45% of students had been physically harassed during the past year due to their sexual orientation. Over one-third had been physically harassed because of their gender expression.

70 *Understanding the Culture of Rural Living*

- Rural students were half as likely to have a gay–straight alliance or other club (27%) addressing LGBTQ issues as urban and suburban students, with over 53%.
- Only 5% of rural students attended schools having comprehensive harassment and assault policies, and one in five (19%) attended schools with no bullying policies of any kind (GLSEN).

Disabled Individuals

Physically Disabled Individuals

According to the US Census Bureau in 2005, over 30% of rural families had one member with a disability, as compared to 28.5% of urban families. People whose disabilities make it difficult to drive can face severe limitations in traveling to work, health-related appointments, and community events. Although the Americans with Disabilities Act (ADA) mandates that public facilities have ramps for easy access for the physically disabled, the cost of building the ramps can be more than an entity can afford. In some cases, the logistics of building wheelchair accessible ramps and bathrooms is a logistical nightmare, particularly in older buildings.

Intellectually Disabled Individuals

Generally speaking, the term intellectually and developmentally disabled (sometimes referred to as delayed) individual refers to a spectrum of disability ranging from what used to be referred to as mentally retarded, or having an IQ of under 70, which ranges from higher functioning people to severe and profound levels as the IQ and functioning level declines. There is also the autistic category of disability, with a spectrum ranging from very high functioning independent people with perhaps some social awkwardness to very low functioning people who need support around the clock. And then there is the category of combined or comorbid mental illness and developmental disabilities. Few mental health professionals are trained in the frequency of this co-occurring combination, and even fewer are competent in treating it. It is thought that an already damaged brain is more susceptible to biochemical imbalances. As research sheds more light on brain activity and function, it is believed more than ever that mental illness is caused by biochemical irregularities.

For centuries, people who are intellectually disabled (ID) have been ostracized and forced to the periphery of society. Unfortunately, standard clinical graduate programs and many medical schools do not include dual diagnosis in their curriculum. To complicate matters, many people with ID have limited communication skills or don't have the emotional awareness or vocabulary to accurately explain how they feel. In addition, the individual's cognitive limitations cause cognitive distortions that make it difficult for the person to determine whether or not they are within the normal realm. Their sometimes limited social exposure further hinders their assessment of themselves. People with ID often have unusual mannerisms such as hand or arm flapping, mouth twitching, pacing, and strange vocalizations such as squealing, which are usually not considered possible symptoms of an emerging mental illness. Among the diagnoses that are common for those in this population include but are not limited to depression, bipolar disorder, schizophrenia, drug addiction, PTSD, and intermittent explosive disorder. For years we have known that people with Down syndrome have a genetic predisposition for early onset dementia, initiating a very different set of needs. We have also known that many with autism have IQs under 70, another form of dual diagnosis. We need to take this kind of approach a step further for all people with ID.

Ironic as it is, a recent study published in *Mother Earth News* in 2015 concluded that pregnant women who live in close proximity to fields and farms where chemical pesticides are applied experience a 66% increased risk of having a child with autism spectrum disorder or developmental delay. Obviously rural areas are the main locations for fields filled with chemicals spread in the name of agriculture. The study, issued by the University of California, Davis, in 2014, stated that although different chemicals have different effects, we need to find ways to reduce pesticide exposure to the general population, but especially to pregnant women. I would add, what about the pesticide residue in the soil from previous years and generations?

The Homeless

Homelessness remains a serious and chronic problem in the United States, according to Manderscheid. He writes that approximately 600,000 people will be homeless tonight, including about 40,000 military veterans. Of this number, between 120,000 and 180,000 (20%–30%) are persons with a serious mental illness. Mental illness is a key risk factor for becoming homeless, and being homeless is a key risk factor for becoming incarcerated. Thus, tonight, about 180,000 persons incarcerated in our county and local jails will be persons with a serious mental illness, many of whom are homeless. Common knowledge in the behavioral health field asserts that if a person does not have a home, then jail becomes their home. It's time we challenged ourselves to figure out how to break this costly and needless cycle of mental illness-homelessness-incarceration.

The Kennedy Forum reports that up to 46% of the homeless population suffers from a severe mental illness and/or substance use disorder. A highly effective solution to homelessness is the Housing First model, which operates under the premise that basic needs like stable housing must be provided before other needs like obtaining a job or addressing behavioral health issues can be successfully addressed.

Some studies and national surveys show that rural homelessness manifests itself differently than urban homelessness. Therefore, different policy approaches and solutions may be needed to lessen and eventually end this issue in America. Rural homeless individuals and families are more likely than their urban counterparts to live with friends or other families, in vehicles, or in temporary housing. The rural homeless population consists of more families rather than individuals (studies show almost 50%); some studies show this population more likely to be working and more likely to be experiencing homelessness for the first time. They are also shown to be less likely to be on government assistance than those in urban areas.

Typically, the word homeless conjures images of people living and sleeping on the streets. The federal government refers to these individuals as "unsheltered" people experiencing homelessness. On the other hand, individuals and families who are considered homeless may also be "sheltered" because they live in shelters, or "doubled-up," or temporarily living with another family or individual. There are several factors that cause housing instability. They include a loss of affordable housing, wages that lag behind the cost of living, unemployment and underemployment, debt that Americans have taken on in order to deal with the above, and the deinstitutionalization of mental health facilities without a corresponding increase in community-based housing and services.

In past years, we dealt with homelessness by getting people off the street and into emergency shelters. Now, Continuums of Care (CoCs), created by the federal Department of Housing and Urban Development—where is the rural in that name?—aim to transition the homeless to a permanent housing solution. These CoCs are tasked with transitioning the homeless through a range of services designed to address the underlying problems and place them in permanent housing that suits their needs. Homelessness in rural areas is often underestimated because many people blend into other households, live in cars or vans, or squat in empty hunting cabins or barns. Counting the number of homeless people in rural areas by counting those in shelters and those living on the street is misleading, because many of these people are not visible to be counted. Those who live in these conditions may have a difficult time applying for and receiving any kind of government aid because they lack a permanent address. Studies have shown that the rural homeless population is less likely to be on government assistance, and this lack of permanent housing may be a large part of the reason why.

The National Alliance to End Homelessness states that almost 50% of the rural homeless population includes children, 37% higher than the national rate. And as with all other rural issues, the infrastructure has less to offer, with the same barriers to treatment such as transportation, isolation, and shortage of services. The pervasive shortage of good quality, affordable housing for both individuals and families remains a huge problem in rural areas. Apartments are extremely difficult to find. The National Advisory Committee on Rural Health and Human Services recommends that in order to better serve the homeless, we need additional flexibility in using existing funding streams to meet the unique needs of rural populations, and to clarify policy guidance on the use of alternate mailing addresses in order to apply for benefits. We also need to encourage each state to follow suit for their programs. More money is needed to launch these projects. When people are stabilized in such housing situations, the opportunity for recovery and returning to productive lives is much greater.

Rural Matters: The First Day of Spring

As I remember it the sound of the crash was deafening. I was leaving a home visit with a client and was focused on getting home for dinner. It was twilight. I noticed there was an unusual number of deer feeding close to the side of the road for this time of year. Dozens of them gathered like tiny communities in various grassy spots along the river. Today is the first day of spring, with the usual snow flurries and ice melting into mud. I beeped the horn several times hoping to scare them off, but one had already begun the lunge toward the driver's side of my car. The long, loud THWAAACK stunned me. I wasn't sure what happened. As I slammed on the brakes, I looked into the rear view mirror to see the deer lying still on the road. I slowly got out of the car to see if she was dead. There was a slight movement in one rear leg, barely discernible, and she was still. Her pale pink tongue hung from the side of her mouth and her wide open eyes vacant. I was thankful she didn't suffer for more than a moment. I recalled the time my dad stopped to comfort a deer struck by the car in front of him. He gently stroked her back until the police came. Seeing how injured she was, they shot her. I looked at the dead deer at the side of the road, struck by her beauty.

It's been snowing on and off all day. Earlier, I slipped on the ice under the snow and landed on my hand. In the moment it took for my feet to slip and my hand to hit the ground, I was aware of free-falling. That second could have been a minute, several minutes, an hour. I felt weightless, not in control of myself. I wondered if the doe felt that timeless, weightless moment before landing on the ground on her side. It is a frozen moment of beauty.

My car was full of dents. White and brown tufts of coarse hair stuck out randomly along with strips of metal trim. Thankfully, the car was still drivable. I paused to take it all in. I was OK, my car was still working, but I took the life of a living thing, intentionally or not. It made me feel sad. I reached into my backpack to get my cell phone, remembering I left it home by accident. I fumbled to remember where the hazard light switch was, and turning it on, I stood near the car to flag someone down. Do I call the police? Can I leave the scene? I should know what to do but I don't, I thought. My mind raced. Several cars sped by. It was the dinner hour, so not much traffic was passing through.

Suddenly, as if out of a dream, a friend I hadn't seen in a while stopped. He pulled the deer further off the road and urged me to move my car farther away from the lane. We used his cell phone to call the state troopers, who said it would be about a half hour before they could get there. It was getting colder and the snow was picking up. After a few minutes we noticed flashing lights further down the road. We walked down together to find a pickup truck stopped after hitting a deer head on. His hazard lights were flashing. The deer had been thrust into the ditch by the side of the road. It was a large buck with 6-point antlers.

It's been a long, cold winter, and now that the snow is melting here in the valley, the deer are coming off the frozen mountaintops to feed. That explains the rash of accidents that have been happening in our area lately. The deer have a ruddy brownish color at this time of year, which blends into the mud that is everywhere. They don't call this mud season for nothing. As time went by, the traffic picked up and several vehicles pulled over to offer help. I saw a coworker I had spoken with earlier in the day, a former client, and another friend, who all took the time to stop and help. Everyone has been hiding from the winter weather for months and is beginning to venture out more. All are glad to see one another, regardless of the circumstance. The company and camaraderie was all we really needed, and to know that our community cared for us. By the time I'd get home, most of town would know what had happened. There would be any number of versions of the story.

A close friend of my daughter's rode by with her family and snapped photos of my damaged car to my daughter. She knew the pickup truck guy because he worked on their family farm. There was talk of asking the police to tag both deer so that they could be taken for food. It hadn't occurred to me that someone could eat the deer. Both dead deer were fair game. As talk of the deer being distributed progressed, I remembered that after bullfights the bull meat is usually donated to a charity or orphanage. A few more cars stopped, and this solemn scene began to feel more like a social gathering. Messages were shouted back and forth across the road: "Don't forget there is an indoor soccer tournament Saturday morning," yelled one woman. "OK, let me know if you need a ride," answered another driver. The messages bounced weightlessly back and forth across the road, while the police lights began to reach us. I gave the policeman my license and registration, and he suggested I wait in the car to stay warm. Usually I carry an extra pair of mittens, a bottle of water, and a book in case of breaking down, but all I had today was the blanket I keep in the trunk. I thought about how hitting a deer has always been my biggest fear about driving these country roads. When I lived near New York City, I thought nothing of picking someone up from the airport late at night, or of driving home from a concert or other event in the middle of the night. But here, here the enemy is a thing of beauty, found in weightless moments on these frosted roads, in this thawing terrain.

References

Affordable Care Act Provisions Affecting the Rural Elderly (ACAPARE). (December, 2011). *National Advisory Committee on Rural Health and Human Services. Retrieved from Alliance for Health Reform. Essentials of Health Policy: A Sourcebook for Journalists and Policymakers.* www.sourcebook.allhealth.org.

Barlett, P. F. (1993). *American Dreams, Rural Realities: Family Farms in Crisis.* Chapel Hill: University of North Carolina Press.

Butler, S. S., & Kaye, L. (2003). *Gerontological Social Work in Small Townsend and Rural Communities.* Binghamton, NY: Haworth Press.

Carr, P. J., & Kefalas, M. J. (2009). *Hollowing Out the Middle: The Rural Brain Drain and What It Means for America.* Boston: Beacon Press.

Carter, R. (2010). *Within Our Reach: Ending the Mental Health Crisis.* Emmaus, PA: Rodale Books.

Centers for Disease Control and Prevention. (2011). *Public Health Action Plan to Integrate Mental Health Promotion and Mental Illness Prevention With Chronic Disease Prevention. 2011–2015.* Atlanta, GA: US Department of Health and Human Services.

Coalition for Mental Health Reform (CMHR). (July 6, 2016). *Concerns with the Helping Families in Mental Health: Crisis Act of 2015—Passed in the House of Representatives.*

Danbaum, D. H. (2006). *Born in the Country: A History of Rural America.* Baltimore: Johns Hopkins University Press.

Dougherty, G., & Mitchell, T. (2011). *Crisis in the American Heartland: Disasters and Mental Health in Rural Environments.* Rocky, MT: DMH Institute Press.

Federal Office of Rural Health Policy (FORHP). (March 17, 2017). *Special Announcement—CDC on Rural Children and Mental Health.*

Grantham, D. (June 1, 2015). National Association of County Behavioral Health and Developmental Disability Directors (NACBHDD). *Under the Microscope: Developing Effective Alternatives to Incarceration for Those With MH and SUD Conditions.* Washington, DC.

Hanson, V. D. (2000). *The Land Was Everything: Letters From an American Farmer.* New York: Free Press.

Homeless in Rural America. (July, 2014). *National Advisory Committee on Rural Health and Human Services.* http://hrsa.gov/advisorycommittee/rural/publications.

Intimate Partner Violence in Rural America. (March, 2015). *National Advisory Committee on Rural Health and Human Services.* http:/hrsa.gov/advisorycommittee/rural/publications.

Joseph, G., Strain, P., & Ostrosky, M. M. (September, 2005). *Fostering Emotional Literacy in Young Children: Labeling Emotions.* Center on the Social and Emotional Foundations For Early Learning. HHS: Child Care and Head Start Bureaus.

Kagan, R., & Schoosberg, S. (1989). *Families in Perpetual Crisis.* New York: W. W. Norton.

Kennedy Forum. (2016). *Navigating the New Frontier of Mental Health and Addiction: A Guide for the 115th Congress.* www.parityregistry.org; www.thekennedyforum.org; www.paritytrack.org.

Kim, N., Mickelson, J., Brenner, B., Haws, C., Yurgelun-Todd, D., & Renshaw, P. (September, 2010). Altitude, gun ownership, rural areas, and suicide. *American Journal of Psychiatry.* www.ncbi.nlm.nih.gov/pmc/articles/PMC4643668/

Manderscheid, R. (August 30, 2016). *Treatment and Housing for Persons With Serious Mental Illness.* www.behavioral.net.

Mental Health and Rural America: 1994–2005. (2005). Washington, DC: Health Resources and Services Administration, Office of Rural Health Policy.

Merritt, J. (April 15, 2015). *How Christians Turned Against Gay Conversion Therapy.* www.theatlantic.com/politics/archive/2015/04/how-christians-turned-against-gay-conversion-therapy/390570.

National Alliance on Mental Illness (NAMI). (July 12, 2016). *We Did It! Mental Health Reform Is Headed to the President's Desk.* www.nami.org.About/NAMI-news/We-Did-It-Mental-Health-Reform-Is-Headed-To-The-Presidents-Desk.

Office of the Surgeon General (US), Center for Mental Health Services (US), National Institute Of Mental Health (US), Rockville (MD), Substance Abuse and Mental Health Services Administration (US). (August, 2001). *Mental Health Care for American Indians and Alaska Natives.*

Olfman, S. (2005). *Childhood Lost.* Santa Barbara, CA: Praeger.

Olfman, S. (2015). *The Science and Pseudoscience of Children's Mental Health.* Santa Barbara, CA: Praeger.

Paceley, M. (July 21, 2016). *Study Determines Needs of LGBTQ Youth in Rural Areas.* www.news.ku.edu/2016/05/06/study-determines-needs-lgbtq-youth-rural-areas-how-social-workers-communities-can-help.

Parental Incarceration's Impact on Children's Health. (May, 2012). The New York Initiative for Children of Incarcerated Parents, The Osborne Association. NYInitiative@osborneny.org.

Perry, M. (2002). *Population: 485, Meeting Your Neighbors One Siren at a Time.* New York: Harper Perennial.

Ramirez-Ferrero, E. (2005). *Troubled Fields: Men, Emotions and the Crisis in American Farming.* New York: Columbia University Press.

Redick, G. (January 5, 2016). *Obama's Executive Actions on Guns Draw Ire of Advocates for Mentally Ill.* Time Warner.

Rhodes, P. (Ed.). (2014). *Mental Health and Rural America.* New York: Nova Science.

Semuels, A. (June 2, 2016). The Greying of Rural America. *The Atlantic.*

Slama, K. (2004). Toward rural cultural competence. *Minnesota Psychologist,* 53(2), 6–13.

Slovac, K., & Singer, M. (February, 2002). Children and violence: Findings and implications from a rural community. *Child & Adolescent Social Work Journal,* 19(1), 35–56.

Smalley, K.B., Yancey, C.T., Warren, J.C., Naufel, K., Ryan, R., & Pugh, J.L. (2010). Rural mental health and psychological treatment: A review for practitioners. *Journal of Clinical Psychology: In Session,* 66(5), 479–489.

Steinbeck, J. (1936). *The Harvest Gypsies.* Santa Clara, CA: Santa Clara University.

Steinbeck, J. (2006) *The Grapes of Wrath.* New York: Penguin Classics.

Sutherland, D. (1998). *The Farmer's Wife.* PBS Home Video.

Taubenheim, A., & Tiano, J. (2012). Rationale and modifications for implementing parent-child interaction therapy with rural Appalachian parents. *Rural Mental Health,* Fall/Winter.

US Census Bureau (2005). www.factfinder.census.gov.

6   Agricultural Roots of Rurality

The agricultural roots of rurality are explored by taking an inside look at the farm crisis, which began in the 1970s and continues today. This chapter examines its causes, results, and possible solutions. It also takes an in-depth look at the farm bill, its makeup, and its effect on farmers and their families. It examines key facts of farming today in the United States and provides famous farming quotes. It takes a look at the suicide increase among farmers, so often the desolate result of losing the family farm. It also provides case studies. Mental illness and substance abuse are re-emerging as their own farming crisis today.

The Farm Crisis

"America discovered the rural crisis in much the same manner as the New World itself was discovered: suddenly and by accident," writes Osha Grey Davidson. On the outside, it appeared that one day American agriculture was galloping along with the highest levels of technology and productivity in the world, and the next day the entire agricultural industry, and therefore the farm population, was in dire straits. Davidson likens the crisis to thinking of the those larger-than-life, mythic farmers who come to mind when we think of our nation's heartland, forever riding combines through fields of ripened grain in our collective imaginations—suddenly showed up on the 6 o'clock news, small and beaten down, choking back tears as the family farm was sold at auction. The farm crisis continues even today.

Our farm population has plummeted from 30 million to 5 million since the 1940s, while the average farm size has more than doubled during the same period. The farm crisis of the 1980s must be viewed as a chapter in the evolutionary story of American agriculture. Rapid technological advancements have profoundly influenced the practice of agriculture throughout the 20th century. These factors are not particular to the United States. They are at work within the context of a global market economy.

Osha Gray Davidson in *Broken Heartland* writes of the farm crisis that in 1979, the United States began an ambitious program to expand the country's agricultural exports. The 1970s saw rising farm incomes and skyrocketing land values. Most assumed that the good times would roll on forever. Banks coaxed farmers to take out larger and larger loans for modernizing and expanding their operations. At first, grain prices slowly declined, losing a penny or two per bushel. Then the decline accelerated. To make up for decreasing profits, farmers were forced to grow more crops. The increased production, in turn, forced grain prices to slide even lower, which in turn led to farmers' putting more land into production, causing trade prices to drop lower still. It was a vicious circle with devastating results for farmers, their families, and their communities. And for those of us on the buying end of the food chain, it cost us more to eat. In October 1979, the Federal Reserve raised the cost of borrowing money. The resulting interest rates threw agriculture and the farmers who practiced it, who had taken on larger amounts of debt, into a wall. At the same time, land values—which are closely tied to commodity prices—started to slide. What is even more frightening is that not only is it a farm crisis, but it is also a crisis of our heartland and the small integrated communities it is made up of. It is a crisis affecting over 90% of our land mass and roughly 20% of our population. That is enormous.

American agriculture is being transformed from a way of life, with a focus on family-owned and operated farms, into a world of agribusiness. There are, however, some significant areas of hope for rural America. These include more alternative fuels; harnessing sun, water, and wind power; the trend toward locally grown foods; natural foods derived from sustainable sources; organic, niche farming, and farm-to-table programs; the desire of many people for the relative safety and security of rural life; and improvements in technology, communications, transportation, and the growth of rural entrepreneurship.

Americans have grown accustomed to the most stable and least expensive food supply of any culture in the history of humankind. Droughts notwithstanding, we have not experienced a major disruption in the food supply in our nation's history.

A large part of our American identity is based on the myths woven into our culture about rural areas and farming in particular. Farmers and their families are known for having a fierce attachment to their land. Our view of rurality has become romanticized to represent a healthier way of life, lived closer to nature and its rhythms rather than the frenetic activity of urban areas. I myself migrated to a rural area from the New York City metropolitan area where I grew up, for some of the very same reasons. Getting back to nature, although trendy at times, is perceived as a wholesome, healthy way to live, as opposed to being a pawn in the industrial/corporate marketplace and subject to the extra stresses of urban life. The farm crisis was both a social and cultural crisis for rural families and communities.

As we've seen, during the 20th century, the rural population of the United States became a shrinking percentage of the total population. In the early 1900s, 60% of the population was rural. Near the end of the century, the rural population had shrunk to about 25%. Here's an astounding statistic: in 1900 farmers accounted for about 40% of the total workforce in the United States, compared to 90% in 1790. By the year 2000, that number would be down to just 1.9%.

Only 6.3% of rural Americans live on farms, and 50% of those families have income from off-farm activities. Even in areas of the country with the highest percentage of farm employment, non-farm employment still accounts for nearly 80% of jobs. In other words, the majority of rural farmers supplement their farm-based income with non-farm employment, whether it's themselves or their family members who work off the farm.

Rural populations can be divided into rural farms and rural non-farms. According to the federal government, a farm is defined as 10 or more acres from which sales of farm products amounted to $50 or more in the preceding tax or calendar year, or a place of fewer than 10 acres from which sales of farm products amounted to $250 or more during the previous year.

The complexity and diversity of attitudes and values Americans have regarding farms is reflected in the language we use to differentiate them: corporate versus non-corporate, family versus non-family, large versus small, organic versus conventional, local versus non-local, industrial versus craft. And in spite of this, we perpetuate the romantic notions we have of the rural life and farming.

In a report about farm accidents traditionally thought to be the leading cause of agricultural fatalities, investigators from the *Tulsa World* and Oklahoma State University made a surprising discovery during the course of their investigation: death certificates from 1983 to 1988 revealed that suicide, rather than accidents, was the leading cause of farm-related deaths. That it has been almost entirely a male phenomenon will probably change as more women become farmers in their own right. The suicide rate among farmers in Oklahoma alone from 1983 to 1989 was three times that of the general population. The prevailing belief is that a man would rather die than admit he's failed.

As farmers accumulated debt, the price of farmland began to rise dramatically. As international demand for grain was met and wheat prices began to level off and eventually fall, many producers found that they were unable to continue to pay for their high-priced land with their agricultural earnings. Farmers were placed in an ironic position: even though their "paper" wealth was expanding, due to the continuing rise in land valuations, they were having cash flow difficulties. This problem was largely solved through the refinancing of debt, a mechanism lenders believed was still viable because of the ongoing increase in the price of land, their principal form of collateral. Farm foreclosures, the financial status of banks, the loss of local businesses, population migration, and even school and hospital closures were the new reality communities had to contend with.

Because the farm crisis has mostly been presented as an economic crisis, very little of the available literature on the psychology of farming and the farm crisis deals with the personal aspect of the crisis, notably land loss and its effects on farm families.

In the restructuring of American agriculture, Yankee entrepreneurs—or agrifarmers as they came to be known—take a more industrial approach to agriculture. They view land as a commodity and farming as a business whose expansion can serve to increase family wealth. Their goal is to effectively and efficiently manage their farm operations to ensure short-term profits. Their farms, consequently, tend to be larger than the average. They deny the more personal aspects that made family farms such a mainstay of rural American culture.

The second kind of denial involved the community. To be labeled by the community as a farmer in financial trouble meant that one was a bad farmer and in effect, a failure. Family-oriented farmers often talked about the lack of decision making ability their more industrial counterparts had.

During the farm crisis, farmers created their own social isolation. Men in crisis would resign from community activities and also from their own families. As a result many men kept to themselves, refusing any offers of help. Others abused chemical substances or began to vent their inner hell through domestic violence, child abuse, and suicide, while other men worked themselves to death. If a woman perceives that her principal responsibility is to be her husband's chief helper, she regards her inability to effectively support him as a failure on her part as well. Both are viewed as moral failings: hers as a wife and homemaker, his as a husband and farmer. High school students spoke to researchers about the unwritten family rules prohibiting discussions of the family's financial troubles outside the home.

When families were forced off their farms, auctions of household items, farm equipment, and tools were publicized in the local newspapers, bulletins, and flyers. To many farmers, this was the ultimate in humiliation. But many families found the silver lining to be an outpouring of support from community members, something the families leaving their farms had not anticipated.

So often, politicians, lawmakers, and government officials who influence rural policy don't acknowledge the dependency urban society has on rural people and places for even their most basic raw materials: food, fiber, and water. And here, our basic source of these resources was experiencing a widespread crisis.

Some believed that the suicide numbers for farmers and their families were dramatically underreported, especially during the farm crisis years. Many of these suicides were written up as heart failure, stroke, or some other sudden onset illness or natural cause. A lot of doctors felt that this would be more beneficial in helping the families, partly because life insurance companies will not pay in the case of suicides. Suicide deaths can be masked as agricultural accidents, and sometimes it is hard to differentiate. The lack of a reported suicide enables families to collect life and health insurance benefits to pay off debts and keep the bank lenders at bay. The majority of farmers associate mental illness with stigma, with many admitting they do not understand mental illness. Most family farmers feel they are the intergenerational keepers of their land, holding the weight of that burden heavy on their shoulders. Even though farm wives owned half of what their husbands owned and did as much work, they were not recognized as a legitimate people in their own right. However, in a great many cases, women's contributions made the difference between foreclosure and the feasibility of staying financially above water.

Cooperative Extension was created through the land grant program of Lincoln's day in order to link advancements in research to the daily lives of rural people through education. This institution has had an immense positive effect on rural areas and has been instrumental in improving the quality of rural life immeasurably.

Whenever a rural manufacturing plant or mine closes, it creates a rural ghetto. In *Broken Heartland*, Osha Gray Davidson writes of the jolt such a severe economic change sets in motion. He writes that it begins a pattern of intergenerational poverty that families have profound difficulty breaking. It touches off a phenomenon in which more prosperous residents move, leaving behind a community in which poverty is even more concentrated. And then the social and economic structure of the rural community adapts to economic shock in ways that accelerate the downward cycle of ghettoization and ultimately cause it to become permanent. Another result is that there is great social and economic pressure in desperate rural communities to look the other way when firms pollute the environment, mistreat workers, or otherwise exploit the area and its resources. He writes that the most insidious part of this process is its self-reinforcing nature, with each downward step making the next one more likely. First farm supply businesses folded, which slowed other businesses. For example, retail sales in Iowa's rural communities slipped an average of 25% in the 1980s. As farms folded, so did the various kinds of businesses and services that had grown up around them.

The Farm Bill

The federal government's farm bill is a law covering numerous aspects of agricultural law, and by extension, opportunities. As an omnibus, or basket of policies, the farm bill is rewritten and renewed about every five years. Although other agricultural laws can be created and passed into law on their own or as attachments to other laws, the farm bill provides a predictable opportunity for lawmakers to address agricultural and food issues in a more holistic way. Since the Great Depression, farm bills have traditionally focused on farm commodity program support for certain staple commodities, typically wheat, cotton, dairy, rice, sugar, corn, and soybeans. In recent years, the farm bill has broadened to include nutritional programs, environmental conservation concerns, forestry, horticulture, bio-energy programs, and a research and Extension Title, which dates back to the Morrill Land Grant Act of 1862, which was established to fund research at land grant institutions.

The most recent farm bill passed in February 2014, and is due to be reviewed and rewritten in 2018. The 2014 bill included 12 titles encompassing commodity price and income supports, farm credit, trade, agricultural conservation, research, rural development, energy, and programs dealing with domestic food and foreign programs. It also included several significant revisions, including income assistance to be provided only in cases of significant yield losses in an area or deep price-based losses. Cotton was eliminated as a program crop, dairy was transitioned to a margin protection program, and livestock producers were given additional protections. Farmers depend greatly on the farm bill contents, as it provides national farm and food policy, but it also stipulates price supports. When Congress stalled in passing the 2012 version, the previous bill expired, leaving no governance document in force for farmers. The headline in a local newspaper at that time was "Locals Wince as Farm Bill Languishes." A Farm Bureau spokesperson stated, "We would hope lawmakers come to their senses and pass something."

Some critics believe that American taxpayers foot the bill for federal farm programs, paying billions every year for farm subsidies, crop deficiency payments, drought disaster aid, and federally funded agricultural research programs. These costs are not counted when agribusiness proponents boast about the nation's plentiful and inexpensive food supply.

We now refer to our society as the 99% of those who struggle economically, and the 1% who rule them. In *Broken Heartland*, Davidson writes about the boarded-up Main Streets and abandoned houses in rural America that are surrounded by huge, thriving agrifarms. Our current system of paying farmers a subsidy for each bushel of grain they produce is a catastrophic flop that leads to overproduction when farmers react by trying to stay afloat by squeezing as much grain out of their land as possible. Davidson continues by suggesting that we adopt a federal farm policy that ensures a stable supply of nutritious and safe food at reasonable prices, protects the environment, and promotes the well-being of the small and medium-sized farms that are the lifeblood of rural communities. What rural America needs, he concludes,

> is not more jobs or money, but more democracy—in the form of citizens willing and able to participate fully in the development and sustenance of their communities. Family farms are essential to making this happen since they are the most invested in their communities.

Most Americans are surprised to learn that largest component of the farm bill is commonly known as food stamps, more recently retitled the Supplemental Nutrition Assistance Program (SNAP). This program was first included in the farm bill in 1973. The largest federal program for rural areas is the farm subsidy program. Rosalynn Carter writes that the change that most of this subsidy goes to large farmers and to corporate or industrial farms is shown by the finding that more than 60% of federal farm subsidy payments go to just 7.2% of the farmers participating in the program. Carter points out that another problem with federal priorities is that although about 90% of rural income is derived from non-farming sources, and agriculture only accounts for about 6% of rural employment, much more federal support goes to farming subsidies than to rural business and community development efforts, which would benefit the majority of people living in rural America.

Other farming laws that affect farmers in all 50 states are the right-to-farm laws that seek to protect qualifying farmers and ranchers from nuisance lawsuits filed by individuals who move into a rural area where normal farming operations exist and who later use nuisance actions to attempt to stop those ongoing operations. Each state has noticeably different content in the specific details of the laws. States' right-to-farm statutes provide the text of each state's laws along with the date of its possible expiration. Generally, right-to-farm laws serve two key purposes. First, they protect farm owners from state and local regulations that might restrict farming, such as burn bans during a drought, because burning is an accepted agricultural practice.

Second, right-to-farm laws protect farmers against the possibility of lawsuits borne of nuisances such as noise from machinery or animals, farm equipment, odors, and other possibly objectionable nuisances. So right-to-farm laws protect farmers against those who move near farmland, only to then complain about all the farming that's going on around them. The laws can also protect new agricultural businesses.

Famous Farming Quotes

Our farmers deserve praise, not condemnation; and their efficiency should be cause for gratitude, not something for which they are penalized.
—President John F. Kennedy

The farmer is the only man in our economy who buys everything at wholesale and pays the freight both ways.
—President John F. Kennedy

Farming looks mighty easy when your plow is a pencil and you're a thousand miles from the corn field.
—President Dwight D. Eisenhower

Burn down your cities and leave our farms, and your cities will spring up again as if by magic; but destroy our farms and the grass will grow in the streets of every city in the country.
—William Jennings Bryan

Whoever makes two ears of corn, or two blades of grass to grow where only one grew before, deserves better of mankind, and does more essential service to his country than the whole race of politicians put together.
—Jonathan Swift

I know of no pursuit in which more real and important services can be rendered to any country than by improving its agriculture, its breed of useful animals, and other branches of husbandman's cares.
—President George Washington
(Farmpolicyfacts.org)

Key Facts on Farming in the United States

- America's farmers not only produce the world's safest and most affordable food and fiber supply, but they also fuel the economy.
- Fewer and fewer farmers are being asked to feed more and more hungry mouths, which won't happen without strong farm policy.
- Nearly 17 million Americans produce, process, or sell food and fiber—9.2% of total US employment.
- US farms and ranches spent $329 billion in local economies to produce $394 billion worth of goods for further processing, consumption, or export in 2012.
- America exported $140.9 billion in farm goods in 2013 with a $37.1 billion trade surplus.
- Americans spend 13% of their income on food—the lowest of any country. This includes money spent at restaurants.
- Farm policy and crop insurance account for only 16% of farm bill funding. Nutrition programs account for 78%.
- Traditional farm support only costs Americans pennies per meal, and on average accounts for roughly one-quarter of 1% of the federal budget.
- If farm policy, including crop insurance, were eliminated today, it would take 100 years to offset the 2012 federal budget deficit alone.
- The world population will grow from 7.2 billion to 9.6 billion by 2050. Farmers will need to double food production by 2050 to keep pace.
- Family farms represent nearly 98% of all US farms and are responsible for 85% of US farm production.
- For every $1 spent on food, farmers receive less than 16 cents for the raw products.
- Net farm income for 2015 is projected to decrease by 32% compared to 2014. Despite tough markets, the 2014 farm bill savings remain intact (www.farmpolicyfacts.org).
- Overall, there was a 16% loss in the total number of farms in New York State from 1983 through 1986, although counting the number of farms lost is a very tricky business because of differing definitions and inadequate data (Fitchen, 1991).
- Delaware County, which changed from largely growing cauliflower to dairy farming, still had nearly 550 commercial farms in 1982, but subsequently lost many farms to a combination of farm problems and strong land-development market for second homes. More Delaware County farms went out through the mechanism of the Federal Dairy Termination Program (the "buyout" or the "whole-herd buyout" of 1986) than was the case in any other county in the state. Nearly 20% of Delaware County's farm operators, or 80 farmers, submitted bids; half of these were accepted (Fitchen, 1991). As of 2012, there were 704 working farms left (http://agcensus.usda.gov) in a rural county larger than the state of Rhode Island and roughly the size of Los Angeles County. By the way, Rhode Island has five counties.

The Critical Need for Affordable Insurance

Rural Americans experience incidence and prevalence rates of mental illness, substance abuse, emotional disturbance, and developmental disability equal to or greater than their urban counterparts. Yet only 25% of the rural poor qualify for Medicaid, compared to 43% of the poor in inner cities (Centers for Medicare and Medicaid Services). Many farm families must send at least one family member off the farm to work somewhere where medical benefits are made available. This has changed some since the birth of the Affordable Care Act (ACA), but farm families often need the income from off-farm sites in order to pay for their insurance and other necessities.

Rural Matters: The Farm Crisis Hits Home

Oh, to be a snail quietly resting on the underside of a frond, hidden away where no one can see me, no one can bother me. No one can upset me but the wind. Flowers bloom all around me, with scents light as clouds, colors bright and pale, spanning the spectrum of emotion.

But I'm not that snail. Not that invisible, although I wish I were. I feel as dark as a thunderhead, the deepest gray of a cloud about to burst. I am about to burst. My farm has been foreclosed on. I have to move myself and my family from the farm that has been in my family for three generations. I am a dark gray failure, golden hay drying in the fields under the hot sun as the bank auctioneer chants his hypnotic song. All the money he raises goes to the bank toward the mortgage and equipment loans. With each item the auctioneer sells, I want to yell out, "It's been good to us, it's a good buy," or "That's my grandfather's saddle, a darn sturdy one. Soft as butter but tough as stone. They don't make them like that anymore." Instead, I look to the horizon and see nothing.

I don't even have time to bale hay for the sale. We cut the hay because the weather report said we'd have more than five dry days. On the fourth day the letter arrived. We've got to be out by Friday morning. That's what the certified letter says. Those bastards, they didn't even have the guts to come out here and tell us themselves that we've got to go. They sent a certified letter signed by some bank president 200 miles away from here. We know the guys over at the Farm Family bank. We've been doing business with them for over 30 years. And they don't even have the decency to sit down with us over a hot cup of coffee and talk straight and in person.

My wife, Margie, is inside packing. In boxes bigger than memories she puts our clothing and living implements. The kids' toys go into another carton. Books and important papers go into yet another. I see tears trickle down her face when she thinks I'm not looking. She wipes them with her sleeve and never stops packing. When she climbs into bed at night and undoes her braid, her long dark hair falls around her like a soft glove. It is then, close-up, that I really see the exhaustion in her eyes. They still shine, but dullness surrounds them. I tell her a funny story to cheer her up. I tell her about the time our new neighbor came by to see the farm and introduce himself. He was taken with the cows and asked which were males and which were females. It was all I could do not to laugh out loud as I told him gently that it stands to reason that only female cows give milk. Margie smiled. The laugh lines around her eyes deepened. She pulled the covers over her and sighed. I put my arm around her as she drifted off to find some peace. Lying there with my eyes closed, I feel their dull heaviness. I slowly grow drowsier, clinging to her for dear life.

I love that woman. We've been together nearly 20 years. We've been through thick and thin together and love each other more than ever. Our kids tease us about kissing each other before one of us leaves the house. It's a ritual we have, like Sunday family suppers and cow-shaped birthday cakes. I hope they get to feel a love as deep as mine and Margie's Above all, I wish that for them. And I hope they remember the farm life with fondness.

I've let Margie down. I wanted to give her everything she wanted. All she wanted was a nice home, a bunch of children, stability, and a decent, wholesome life. I've let everyone down. My children, my parents, my aunts and uncles, and cousins. And more than anyone, I've let myself down.

When the trucks pulled up yesterday to haul the cows away, I cried. I couldn't help myself. I'd been holding it all in through months of worrying and plotting to avoid this day. I'd sit up alone late at night, the living room as dark as the hide of a heifer. Every once in a while I'd let a few tears slip because I was alone, but I couldn't talk to anyone about any of my worries because I love them too much to have them worrying along with me. Even my friends. Most of them have the same worries. The drought is what dried us all up. That, politics and policies—tangled as knotweed.

You see, about five years ago, farming was actually a mildly profitable thing to be doing. A fine, honorable profession it is, a highly spiritual one too. But before that, it was often a money-losing thing. Then the government made trade agreements with the Soviet Union and other countries for us to export more grain than ever, and it became profitable to grow grain on the extra acreage we have. With the profits, many of us decided to reinvest them into our farms by buying the newfangled farm machinery that came on the market. Oh, the salesmen promised us it would streamline our productivity like a high-speed railway going from Albany to New York. They promised we could cut our planting time, our harvesting time, and our expenses by using their equipment and hiring fewer migrant workers. They promised those darned machines would cut our milking time, freeing us up to do all the other chores a farmer has got to do in order to run a farm smooth as a river rock. So many of me and the other farmers signed on to loans as large as the biggest barns, feeling optimistic about our futures.

But they lied. Oh, those machines cut our labor time all right. They weren't lying about that part. What they lied about was the future of the institution called family farming. They knew that so many of the farms that had been foreclosed on were taken over by the large agribusiness corporations. Some families were allowed to remain living on the farms and work for the corporations. They ended up feeling like slaves did before the Civil War. They owned nothing, and did what they were told. In return, they got to stay on the land they loved. I wonder if it was worth it. Maybe it's better to move on like the clouds do on a windy day. Moving and drifting, unaware of where they are headed. At some point, I figure a man's got to cut his losses. You know, like having a stillborn calf. You can't just always stand around crying in your beer. Well, I guess you can, but it sure doesn't change a thing.

The situation with all us farmers foreclosing is clear as mud. We were taken for a ride when the government decided to put a trade embargo on the Soviet Union and all the grain we grew that year had nowhere to go. Like a large tree fallen into the river so the water has nowhere to go, my oats and everyone else's sat in mountains of doom. The granary even had to lay off a dozen guys because there just was no place for that darn grain to go. All that wheat, alfalfa, corn for meal, and barley, well it all just rotted in the rain. No one had much income that year. The only income we had was from the milk, and that just wasn't enough to get us all fed and clothed and kept warm, because the government set the price for milk so low it was worse than a bad joke. We managed, but this time is different. It sure is different.

Russell Gulliver, he hanged himself in his barn when everyone thought he was out there milking the cows. His oldest son found him hanging there like strange fruit, as the song goes. The strangest and saddest fruit any of us ever saw. Wordless and wide-eyed, the kid pointed helplessly toward the barn as me and the others arrived one by one and came running out of our cars. We had to get on a high ladder to cut him down that night. That was a dark moonless night all right. His son just about fainted by the time we all got there, he just stood there like a statue with his eyes wide and his mouth open, but no words could get out. They were trapped inside him. And Russ isn't the only one who took the easy way out. There are plenty of them in all parts of this large county they call Delaware. I don't know them but I'm sad for them just the same. Who says it couldn't have been me who took that route. Instead, I'm listening to the wasp-like drone of the auctioneer and wishing I was a snail wallowing peacefully on the underside of a frond.

The farm crisis continues today in different forms. Environmental stressors facing today's farmers are related to climate change, and are likely to worsen rather than reverse themselves. Examples are all over America—the most severe outbreak of tornadoes and stronger hurricanes are happening in record numbers, extreme droughts like the recent one in California, heavier than usual snowfall in the northern and eastern states all make farming more difficult and unpredictable. In a population with such deep connections to their land, with family connections that run even deeper, and where firearms are easily accessible, mental illness is re-emerging as its own farming crisis.

References

Addressing Mental Health Workforce Needs in Underserved Rural Areas: Accomplishments and Agriculture is Vital to New York's Economy. (2015). Overland Park, KS: National Crop Insurance Services.

Bagalman, E. (2016). *The Helping Families in Mental Health Crisis Reform Act of 2016.* Washington, DC: Congressional Research Service.

Barlett, P. F. (1993). *American Dreams, Rural Realities: Family Farms in Crisis.* Chapel Hill: University of North Carolina Press.

Brown, D. L., & Schafft, K. (2011). *Rural People and Communities.* Malden, MA: Polity Press.

Brown, D., & Swanson, L. (Eds.). (2003). *Challenges for Rural America in the Twenty-First Century.* University Park: Pennsylvania State University Press.

Carter, R. (2010). *Within Our Reach: Ending the Mental Health Crisis.* Emmaus, PA: Rodale Books.

Census.gov/geo/tiger/glossry2.html.

Centers for Medicare and Medicaid Services. www.cms.gov.

Childs, A. W., & Melton, G. B. (1983). *Rural Psychology.* New York: Plenum Press.

Cloke, P., Marsden, T., & Mooney, P. H. (Eds.). (2006). *Handbook of Rural Studies.* Thousand Oaks, CA: Sage.

Davidson, O. G. (1996). *Broken Heartland: The Rise of America's Rural Ghetto.* Iowa City: University of Iowa Press.

Fitchen, J. (1991). *Endangered Spaces, Enduring Places.* Boulder, CO: Westview Press.

Flora, C. B., & Flora, J. L. (2008). *Rural Communities, Legacy and Change* (3rd ed.). Philadelphia, PA: Westview Press/Perseus Books.

Goldman, H. H., Buck, J. A., & Thompson, K. S. (2009). *Transforming Mental Health Services: Implementing the Federal Agenda for Change.* Arlington, VA: American Psychiatric Association.

Goldschmidt, W. (1978). *As You Sow.* New York: Allanheld, Osmun.

Hanson, V. D. (2000). *The Land was Everything: Letters From an American Farmer.* New York: Free Press.

Harrington, M. (1997). *The Other America.* New York: Scribner.

Imhoff, D. (2012). *Food Fight: The Citizens Guide to the Next Food and Farm Bill.* Healdsburg, CA: Watershed Media.

Kagan, R., & Schlosberg, S. (1989). *Families in Perpetual Crisis.* New York: W.W. Norton.

National Center for Farmworker Health. *Farmworker Health Factsheets.* May, 2013.

Parental Incarceration's Impact on Children's Health. (May, 2012). The New York Initiative for Children of Incarcerated Parents, The Osborne Association. NYInitiative@osborneny.org.

Perry, M. (2002). *Population 485, Meeting Your Neighbors One Siren at a Time.* New York: Harper Perennial.

Ramirez-Ferrero, E. (2005). *Troubled Fields: Men, Emotions and the Crisis in American Farming.* New York: Columbia University Press.

Sawyer, D., Gale, J., & Lambert, D. (2006). *Rural and Frontier Mental and Behavioral Health Care: Barriers, Effective Policy Strategies, and Best Practices.* Washington, DC: National Association for Rural Mental Health.

A Short History and Summary of the Farm Bill. (2016). Arlington, VA: Farm Policy Facts. www.farmpolicy.org.

Smalley, K. B., Warren, J., & Rainer, J. (Eds.). (2012). *Rural Mental Health: Issues, Policies, and Best Practices.* New York: Springer.

Steinbeck, J. (1936). *The Harvest Gypsies.* Santa Clara, CA: Santa Clara University.

Steinbeck, J. (2006). *The Grapes of Wrath.* New York: Penguin Classics.

Sutherland, D. (1998). *The Farmer's Wife.* PBS Home Video.

Wood, R. E. (2008). *Survival of Rural America: Small Victories and Bitter Harvests.* Lawrence: University Press of Kansas.

7 Disaster Mental Health

This chapter delves into two types of disasters—natural and man-made—and the effect they have on mental health for individuals, families, and communities. Their symptoms, treatment options, and patterns of behavior are explored, as well as short-term versus long-term effects. With the increase in severe storms such as hurricanes and blizzards, large numbers of damaging tornadoes, record-setting forest fires, earthquakes, floods, mudslides, and other climatic events becoming the norm, it is more important than ever that we ensure that crisis counseling is available in rural areas where there are fewer resources available for recovery. It is critical that trauma-informed practitioners be available because most of these adverse weather crises occur in rural areas.

While it is beyond the scope of this book to go deeply into trauma, post-traumatic stress disorder (PTSD), and the psychological consequences of disasters, it is certainly worth mentioning the many kinds of natural disasters that can ravage an area. In rural areas, we know that resources are fewer and need to be spread even thinner than they are normally. We also know that the effects of a terrorist attack, public health emergency, or natural disaster can be long-lasting. The resulting trauma affects both those directly affected by the disaster as well as those not directly affected. There is a natural progression of emotions most people go through after experiencing a disaster, and the majority has symptoms that gradually fade with little further intervention needed. These symptoms include but are not limited to disorientation; difficulty communicating and concentrating; becoming easily frustrated; feeling depressed, sad, or hopeless; having headaches and/or stomach aches; difficulty sleeping; crying easily; feeling overwhelming guilt or self-doubt; fears of crowds or of being alone; and an intense reluctance to leave home.

Equally important is that just as an individual goes through a continuum of emotions, so do communities. Immediately after the impact of an event, the community is in the throes of a heroic phase in which all are taking stock of the situation and reacting to help return the community to safety. As safety is put into place, the community becomes highly cohesive, akin to a honeymoon phase. People are helping each other, crying together, sharing whatever resources they can, and feeling that they are in it together as a community.

In my own experience in living through several "hundred-year" floods and blizzards, before we had a local radio station, if we wanted to get local news we had to turn to a station located about 40 minutes away. Often that station ran on taped music segments that might run for an hour or more. There is often a huge difference in weather between here and there, making those reports unreliable. For the first 15 years I lived in this rural upstate New York area, 911 emergency service didn't exist. If the county closed the roads, there was little way to find out. It is still that way in many rural areas in America, with no reliable internet or cell phone service.

Natural Disasters

Weather is the great leveler of the fields in rural lands. The old adage in my home town is, "If you don't like the weather, wait 10 minutes." And many are the times I headed out to work in the winter only to have a snow squall pass through and quickly dump several inches of slick snow and ice onto the road before the sun comes out, as if by a light switch.

In the 26 years I have lived in rural upstate New York, we have experienced three hundred-year floods. By the time you read this, we may have experienced a fourth. The first was from the fast melting of over 3 feet of snow during the typical January thaw. The second was a fourth of July rainstorm that dropped 5 or 6 inches of rain in a few morning hours. The third was from Hurricane Irene, which devastated the area, washing away homes, bridges, downing trees and power lines, and flooding the entire region. Roads in several counties were officially closed, meaning that anyone driving on them did so at their own risk. It is not uncommon for homes to be without cell service or without a telephone at all. Rescue workers from out of town can find it difficult to locate people when the directions given are to turn right after the second red barn.

Other kinds of natural disasters that impact rural areas include high winds, volcanic eruption, floods, droughts, forest fires, mudslides, sinkholes, earthquakes, tornadoes, severe thunderstorms and blizzards, ice storms, tsunamis, and explosions.

Quite often in rural areas, the only option for mental health services is a public or community mental health facility. Yet well over half of the US population lives in designated psychiatric shortage areas, making it critical for qualified counselors to be able to come from other areas. Local counselors and mental health professionals need to be brought together along with any school administrators, social workers, health care workers, and even clergy and firemen to help with the initial plan formulation. Caregivers will need support and debriefing at regular intervals, which can be done by the out-of-town team members. Flyers should be created that outline existing resources and the extended resources being brought to the disaster area. Plans should be made to have offices set up in a central location. Public education can be provided to civic and business groups, while public service announcements about where to find help should be in newspapers, newsletters, radio, television, and social media.

Disaster aides would do well to check in with the local sites where business is often conducted, such as farm organization meetings, Cooperative Extension offices, luncheonettes, and town halls and firehouses. Here they can connect to the local level of crisis workers, those with the largest stake in the whole affair because it is their home. Crisis counseling will need to take many forms and happen in many different settings, including barns, granges, churches, and farm kitchens. Some of those who are sifting through the rubble of what was their own home may need to be seen on their property.

Of the qualifications needed in a crisis counselor, the most important besides empathy are adaptability and open-mindedness. Doherty points out that in the current times of crisis, it is critical that mental health professionals in rural areas become aware of recent research, training, and approaches to crisis intervention, traumatology, compassion fatigue, disaster mental health, critical incident stress management, post-traumatic stress, and related areas.

One community-based institution that disaster counselors will want to tap into is schools, which have their finger on the pulse on their rural communities. Counselors can connect with school assemblies; individual, small, and large group counseling; and other school-based activities such as running classroom activities, after-school activities, or clubs. Appropriate activities include but are not limited to students creating disaster kits, disaster-related coloring books, poster contests, art therapy, music therapy, skits, service learning projects, and writing and illustrating poems, stories, or articles about their experiences.

The vast majority of children who experience a natural disaster are physically and emotionally healthy children who need help returning to their normal equilibrium. With families, the main role of the crisis counselor is to give its members permission to share their feelings with each other as well as with others. Family members might need help in realizing that what they are feeling is normal given the shock of the situation. It is common for parents to recognize signs of trauma and behavioral changes in their children before realizing it in themselves. Common reactions after the disaster may include any of the following:

* Trouble sleeping/fatigue/nightmare
* Flashbacks/recurrent dreams
* Crying easily, short attention span
* Change in appetite/headaches
* Increase in interpersonal conflicts
* Refusal to attend school

* Anxiety, social withdrawal, confusion
* Disruption of work, school, and social activities
* Somatic complaints that are unfounded
* Preoccupation with the event
* Feelings of despair, guilt, depression, anger
* Questioning spiritual beliefs

* Uncontrolled mood swings
* Apathy, isolation, and detachment
* Use of drugs or alcohol to avoid the issues at hand
* Rage, often focused on those helping.
* Shame over vulnerability

Schools can be of significant help to children in recovery from disaster. According to Dougherty, many school administrators have a catch-22 attitude regarding post-crisis debriefing. Some believe it only creates more anxiety and disturbance in the school. Some research shows that the opposite is true. The anxiety and related energy levels of children in disaster-affected areas often result in various levels of chaos if not given an appropriate and productive outlet. Such in-school services can make the difference between children developing PTSD and those who are helped early enough in the process that they recoup themselves and move on.

The methodology for successful crisis counseling involves establishing a rapport; identifying, defining, and focusing on the problem; understanding and validating feelings; listening carefully; and communicating clearly. It is also important for crisis counselors to address the steps forward in realistic terms, including the estimated time of ending temporary housing to either return home or start living in a new home. Learned helplessness can occur in disaster situations, especially those that drag on for many months or longer. Because most humans are spiritual beings in some way or another, it is critical for a crisis counselor to help the individual(s) involved to find meaning in some kind of outcome of the disaster, minimize feelings of helplessness, and inspire a sense of being in command of or having mastery over themselves and their situation. If these remain unresolved, a lifetime of depression, anxiety, and a host of other emotional and physical disorders can result.

Dougherty writes that when the event is perceived realistically, there is an awareness of the connection between the event and the feeling of stress. Any attempt to resolve the problem will be affected accordingly. When the perception of the event is distorted, there is no awareness between the connection between the event and the feeling of stress. It is critical to identify what meaning the event has in the victims eyes.

As in Gestalt therapy, where an individual is helped back to a state of homeostasis, a trauma response that fails to meet this goal becomes unresolved trauma. This reaction is at the far end of the spectrum of emotions and can cause the nervous system to run amok, which in turn can cause permanent psychological and even physical damage.

Most elderly residents take life-perpetuating prescription medications, which can be impossible to find during a disaster in a rural area. Anyone of any age who takes prescription medication should have at least an extra week's worth on hand at any given time. A crisis counselor seeking low-income community members may have to look hard, because they are often difficult to locate. A lack of stability in their lives regarding living arrangements, employment and social connections, and the higher level of need than predisaster tends to make their situations overwhelming.

As we've seen with the record-breaking hurricanes of 2017, the full impact of a disaster in any area may not be known for quite a few months. For example, in agricultural areas, a flood may seem even more devastating in the fall with the absence of a harvest. The impact a crisis can have in an agricultural area ranges from the immediate housing and animal needs to the erosion of topsoil, increased contaminants, and a sharp increase in food prices nationwide. Farmers who do apply for federal assistance early on may grossly underestimate their need because of these factors. And as we know, asking for help to begin with is very difficult for this population that lives in a culture of self-reliance and independence.

To complicate counseling strategies, many social scientists believe that all human beings hold some form of spiritual belief. In fact, in most rural areas, people have a strong spiritual connection to nature, to the land, growing food, raising animals, and being part of a community of mostly like-minded folks. Through the centuries, all kinds of rituals have been brought to light regarding planting, harvesting, birth, death, physical and religious or other spiritual issues, and nationalism. So many of these beliefs and rituals are embedded in rural cultures and form the backbone of the community. The religious traditions have become the primary expression of their sense of right and wrong, moral versus immoral, and good versus bad in many rural areas. Like Kübler-Ross's stages of grief, the phases of a disaster often overlap and are not necessarily experienced in the order presented. Dougherty writes that the phases of a disaster are:

- Warning or Threat Phase.
- Impact Phase: characterized by confusion and disorganization.
- Rescue or Heroic Phase: need for connection to local organizations as well as crisis counselors.
- Remedy or Honeymoon Phase: needs assessment is started and a structure for mental health disaster response is laid out.
- Inventory Phase: disaster workers are becoming tired and possibly burned out. This is the time when plans to close programs begin. Often the red tape of bureaucracy feels insurmountable.
- Disillusionment Phase: victims often feel estranged from others, disoriented because their communities are permanently altered. The initial feeling of coming together has worn off as the anniversary date looms with that date having the potential for bringing strong feelings back to the surface.
- Recovery Phase: life moves on as the disaster recedes.

The key word to keep in mind during disasters is change. Because the situation is fluid and ongoing, any attempt to help needs to be dynamic in order to be effective. Another key thought is that much of the angst of dealing with a disaster depends on an individual's personal interpretation of the event. Because we humans need to find meaning in our experiences, it is critical to help a person find their meaning in the crisis. If the meaning a person discovers can lead to a shift from victim to survivor can make a huge difference in the quality and speed of recovery. By extension, the speed and extent to which parents recover directly impacts the psychological recovery of their children.

Children are in particular need of mental health interventions after disasters for many reasons. While they may experience the same reactions as adults, they are less experienced at dealing with stress, they have less emotional literacy and vocabulary to articulate their feelings, they are dependent upon adults, and particularly in a rural area they may know others who were injured or killed. Additionally, during a crisis, parents may be more preoccupied with dealing with the logistics of salvaging a home, its contents or the like, and therefore may be less available to children. Many farm kids know that they will be expected to help with disasters on the farm, which may mean missing school and other activities important to them.

When the dust has settled, it is important for crisis counselors to set up community events. By this time, the honeymoon period is over and the reality and perhaps permanency of the situation has set in. These events can be anything from a community picnic to an interfaith service or some form of entertainment as a diversion. Not everyone will be ready for this, as we all grieve at our own pace, but for those who are ready these events can provide education, closure, and inspiration for moving forward while fostering close community connections. When the anniversary date of the event arrives, it may unsettle the emotions of many who thought they had reached the other side. Such an event around this date may be a way to have the community come together again to celebrate their rebuilding efforts and reconnect as a community.

As we've seen in the farm crisis, when disaster strikes the agricultural community, all businesses related to farming suffer as well. Grocery stores and other food markets, restaurants, clothing stores, and other kinds of retailers take an economic plunge. Like any other disaster, the full impact may not be known for months. Farmers, post-disaster, have to deal with its impact on the planting and harvesting season, the erosion of invaluable topsoil, contaminants as from a flood, and fluctuations in market prices. Thus, there is the strong possibility that following a disaster in a heavily agricultural area, there may very well follow an economic crisis. To compound the disaster further for farmers, there are time limits on applying for assistance, and they may not know up front if assistance is needed. Many farmers have an innate distrust of government or outsiders, which, coupled with the cultural hesitancy to ask for or accept help, the prospect of dealing with bureaucracy, mountains of paperwork and red tape, further deepens the crisis for them.

Man-Made Disasters

Man-made disasters include but are not limited to plane crashes, terrorist incidents, chemical spills or leaks, and nuclear reactor malfunctions. I would argue that there is a fine line between natural and man-made disasters. For example, recent earthquakes in Oklahoma are known to be caused by fracking.

Dougherty writes that when stress originates externally, it causes internal changes. Certain events can cause a strong emotional reaction in one person and leave another indifferent. Crisis counseling programs play a very important role in helping rural families to assess the issues involved in a disaster and make good decisions regarding their immediate and long-term needs. With the recent record-breaking hurricanes in Houston and Florida, this became very apparent.

There are many other considerations for mental health during a disaster. At a minimum, regional licensing reciprocity during a crisis or disaster is needed that would allow all licensed categories of mental health providers to participate in the aftermath and healing. For example, if during Hurricane Sandy mental health practitioners from New Jersey's neighboring states of Pennsylvania, Delaware, New York, and Connecticut were able to help the relief effort without having to worry about licensing constraints, there would have been an overabundance of qualified mental health professionals available to help out. In addition, we need to include psychotropic medications in emergency stockpiles of medications. And we need to do a better job of paying attention to the mental health needs of first responders. These brave people are often the victims of vicarious or secondary trauma.

References

Dougherty, G., & Mitchell, T. (2011). *Crisis in the American Heartland: Disasters and Mental Health in Rural Environments*. Rocky, MT: DMH Institute Press.
Herman, J. (1997). *Trauma and Recovery: The Aftermath of Violence From Domestic Abuse to Political Terror*. New York: Basic Books.
Levine, P. (1997). *Waking the Tiger: Healing Trauma*. Berkeley, CA: North Atlantic Books.
Levine, P. (2010). *In an Unspoken Voice: How the Body Releases Trauma and Restores Goodness*. Berkeley, CA: North Atlantic Books.
Schorr, L.B., with Schorr, D. (1988). *Within Our Reach: Breaking the Cycle of Disadvantage*. New York: Anchor Books.
Van der Kolk, B. (2015). *The Body Keeps the Score: Brain, Mind and Body in the Healing of Trauma*. New York: Penguin.

8   Poverty

Poverty is a constant in rural life and can become intergenerational. The connection between poverty and mental illness is well documented. This chapter surveys the effects that high poverty levels have on rural communities, individuals, and families. Some of the effects are school consolidations, empty storefronts and malls, depopulation, workforce shortages, leaning silos, and dilapidated barns. Needs assessments are a highly viable way of gauging a community's needs. The Substance Abuse and Mental Health Services Administration's (SAMHSA's) Strategic Prevention Framework is presented as a reliable, free comprehensive tool that can be used in assessment. A case study is included.

Poverty Is a Constant in Rural Life

- Over 25% of rural workers earn less than the federal poverty rate.
- Child poverty is also higher in rural areas, with more than half of all rural children (3.2 million) living in poverty in female-headed households.
- Children of color are of particular risk, with 46.3% of rural African American children, 43% of rural Native American children, and 41.2% of rural Hispanic children living in poverty.
- During the 1990s, several million people exited the city seeking life in the country, representing a rural migration trend that contrasts with the rural-to-city out-migration trends of the early and mid-20th century. We are still experiencing a depopulation phenomenon today.

Rural counties still have poverty rates almost 25% higher than urban counties and account for almost 90% of all the "persistent poverty" counties, defined by the US Department of Agriculture as counties that have experienced poverty rates above 20% for the past 30 years.

According to Smalley, Warren, and Rainer in *Rural Mental Health and Psychological Treatment: A Review for Practitioners*, the connection between poverty and mental health is one of the best established in psychiatric epidemiology. Two consistent symptoms across most rural populations are poverty and the inability to access affordable mental health services. An estimated 17% of adult rural residents live below the federal poverty line, as compared with 14% of urban residents. Poverty rates are even higher for minority rural residents. The poor tend to experience longer periods of time without health insurance and are less likely to seek care when they can't pay because of pride and the lack of sliding scale services in rural areas.

One important contributing factor is that there is a common pattern of serial monogamy that is more prevalent in rural areas. For example, a woman living with one man for a considerable period of time, bearing his children, and then moving on to another man and perhaps bearing a child of his. Indeed, I have worked with siblings, as many as four with four different fathers. In many cases the children are very close in age, such as four children aged 6 and under in one family.

Rural decay began decades ago when railroads and interstate highways bypassed towns, a rival community became the county seat, or school districts merged to a regional model, leaving villages no choice but to close schools. What we are seeing now in many rural areas across the country are the later stages of decay, such as the boarded-up shops and empty storefronts, abandoned and decaying housing, broken-down cars in yards, huge collapsed barns, and silos listing to one side. Notice that we refer to pockets of the formerly thriving industrial Midwest as the Rust Belt. If not attended to, the forest will reclaim the land, as it has reclaimed so many farm fields. Many rural towns have creatively flaunted their "historic character," as a way of marketing themselves for economically dependable urbanites to vacation there, buy country homes, and boost the local, often failing economy. When the urbanites arrive, however, they are shocked to find that many rural areas do not have cell phone service, high-speed internet, or many other modern conveniences they have come to rely on.

An issue that is becoming more common in small towns is the consolidation of local schools in favor of regional schools. Most rural schools have "central" schools containing grades K-12 in one building. As the population shrinks, it becomes harder to justify keeping small schools open with the appropriate number of faculty and staff. Absent from most discussions of rural school consolidation is any consideration of the long-term and often devastating economic and social effects of school consolidations and closings on the communities themselves. First there is the loss of jobs to factor in, and then you have to consider that children from grades K-12 will now face longer bus rides, sometimes well in excess of an hour each way. Schools are most often the largest employers in rural towns, and it is not easy to re-employ oneself with an equivalent job. Often this necessitates moving to another area or commuting long distances in order to survive financially. I have had to do the latter for many years. Many, many people are underemployed—I know landscapers with master's degrees in business, librarians with doctorates in English literature, and bartenders who are former managers from large corporations.

Most of the growth in rural areas can be attributed to improved transportation and advances in agricultural technology. Wood writes in *The Survival of Rural America* that most rural communities reached their population peak between 1900 and 1950, before the interstate highway system was built and before large-scale farming entered the picture. In the mid-century, the location of rural towns was determined by the distance a person could walk or ride his horse in a few hours, which meant that towns sprang up every few miles, usually 10, give or take a few. Later, towns developed around rivers, then railroads, then eventually highways, which in turn influenced town growth and survival. The result has been that many towns were created to service needs, such as railroads, and have suffered the unintended consequences of progress in transportation.

Wood points out that during the 1960s until the 1980s, when the decline of the family farm began to take its toll, most thought that the depopulation rural communities were experiencing was a temporary phenomenon. Those with blinders on thought that the population losses were just a correction or adjustment to the artificial overpopulation that had been induced by government stimulation through programs like the 1862 Homestead Act. This theory maintained the idea that rural towns would lose population. But a stable population proved to be an impossibility, and by the year 2000 it was clear that depopulation was not a passing phase, that in fact there was nothing to prevent small towns from unincorporating or disappearing entirely. Some small towns in my area have done just that out of necessity. Along with the consequences of a shrinking population in rural areas is the smaller share of federal government representation and government funding that is tied to population numbers, making help harder to find.

As of 2007, Kansas and Oregon were the only states to have created dedicated rural development offices independent of the existing governmental structure. Such programs help increase the visibility of rural communities, help them to establish their identities, and better enable them to have their needs considered in a broader context than simply as extensions of a state's agricultural policies.

Needs Assessments in Rural Areas

Needs assessments are valuable tools to help gather information for use for in program development, planning for the future, and determining what subpopulations need to be reached.

Needs assessments are used to identify current community conditions and issues, the subgroups affected by them, and what, if any, resources are available to address the problem. The information gathered should be shared with the population afterward in order to deepen their understanding and encourage them to buy into being stakeholders. One use for the information is for possible funders. Collaboration is the name of the game in the funding world, with good reason.

Although there are many models for conducting needs assessments, the Substance Abuse and Mental Health Services Administration's (SAMHSA's) Strategic Prevention Framework (SPF) is a comprehensive guide to plan, implement, and evaluate problems. The SPF is a planning process for preventing substance abuse that helps assess epidemiological data, including the consequences of substance misuse and consumption patterns, resources, and readiness to address identified problems. It utilizes five steps and two guiding principles to offer a comprehensive process for addressing the substance misuse and related behavioral health problems facing their communities. The effectiveness of the SPF begins with a clear understanding of community needs and involves community stakeholders in all stages of the planning process. The steps of the SPF include:

1. *Assess needs.* What is the problem, and how can I learn more?
2. *Build capacity.* What resources to I have to work with? This involves building and mobilizing local resources and readiness to establish and maintain a prevention system, and needs people with motivation and willingness to commit local resources.
3. *Plan.* What needs to be done and how should I go about it?
4. *Implement.* How can I put my plan into action?
5. *Evaluate.* Is my plan succeeding?

Guiding principles include a strong emphasis on interacting effectively with diverse populations and aspiring to sustainability and long-term results. The SPF is data driven, and it is dynamic in that it is designed to be circular rather than a linear model—as the needs of a community change, and as resources become more plentiful, it should be repeated.

The resource section in the back of this book can be used for further information. In particular, the Rural Health Information Hub is a wealth of information about rural issues, statistics and resources (www.ruralhealthinfo.org). In addition, local sources for statistical and trend information include town and county vital records such as social services, public health, law enforcement agencies, hospitals and health care, professional journals, and websites. The SAMHSA website for free tools for conducting needs assessments (http://capt.collaboration.edc.org) is part of their Center for the Application of Prevention Technology.

Rural Matters: What Defines Life?

On a damp, cold, winter afternoon she slowly climbed the steps to the office. I gave her a warm hello and she grunted something that may have been hello back. In her arms clutched tightly to her chest was Teddy, her stuffed bear. Her short, dark hair highlighted an angelic face and dark brown eyes. It was often hard to see her eyes because they were always downcast, the corners of her mouth turned down to match. She was 5 years old and had just started kindergarten.

She was not allowed to see her father, who recently returned home from jail. The order of protection against him was still in effect. He had started dealing crack cocaine because he needed the money. His girlfriend and baby mama was covered in bruises, eggplant-hued spots on her arms, her collarbone and her left eye. The midsections of her arms had marks from his hands and throbbed as she cried out. He was in a jealous rage because another guy gave her a wink. "It wasn't my fault," she yelled in defense. "I didn't do anything to encourage him to do that." Life in a small town can be like living in a glass house, but someone put a crack in the roof. It tumbled down, glistening in the flickering red and blue police lights. The silver handcuffs caught the light in the otherwise dark night. A flicker of white in his eyes showed a defiant expression. "I didn't do nothing," she heard him yell through the night air. The cold of numbness scared her as she lay under the covers. She got up to look out the window. Neighbors also heard the yelling and screaming and called the police. Upon arrival, they searched the house and found his stash, which was not well hidden in the basement.

The flashing lights were startling, but not as frightening as the yelling, cursing, and sporadic crashing sounds as her mother was thrust from one side of the living room to the other. She had crept quietly out of her room to see what all the noise was about, but when she saw her mother reeling from being pushed, heard her sobs and screams, she ran back to her room and hid under the covers holding on to her Teddy for dear life. She wondered if he would come into the darkness to find her and hit her. She didn't understand why he acted like that, but it wasn't the first time. He could be so much fun to be around, teaching her how to fish, how to play softball, even how to build a rock wall. She never could relax completely, however, always afraid of making him angry. "I can't make him mad at me," she would think. "If he gets mad at me, he'll hurt me. He did one time. He spanked me so hard with a belt, it left red marks on my back that stung and burned. I don't ever want that to happen again. Anything to keep him happy. We can't afford to live anywhere else. Mom stays home with me. How would we get food and clothes? Who would take care of us?" She felt panicked and her breathing was rapid. Like bellows to a fire, her emotions took over, fanning the flames of shock and disbelief.

Even now she has so much anger locked inside herself. Like the stuffing inside Teddy, it starts to feel solid. Stuffed there like wadded old cotton rags, one upon the next and the next until there are many layers of protection. It's easier to feel nothing than to feel the pain she knew from that life. That kind of pain is the rust of life, the corrosion of trauma, the oxidation of early aging.

After he was taken away to jail, she heard the familiar rusty creak of the front door. She got up, clutching Teddy tightly, and tiptoed in to find her mom sprawled out on the couch sobbing. The flashing lights were gone and the room was mostly dark, save for a small night light in the bathroom. She couldn't see the bruises, the cuts and scrapes; they would not be real for her until morning's light. She softly said, " Mommy, mommy, are you okay?" At first her mother couldn't hear her, so she repeated herself louder. The sobbing slowed like a receding wave, and she ran over, arms outstretched, Teddy falling to the wayside.

She sat down in my office, refusing to take her coat or boots off. She sat holding Teddy looking downward. He was her stability, her strength, and her protector. His look was startling. Teddy had no hair left. She had anxiously pulled it all off. Poor Teddy was stark naked, but he was her everything. What defines life is motion in the center of our bodies. She saw that in Teddy's bald body. She told me, "If you look at him hard enough, and believe in him enough, you will see it too."

References

Bird, D.C., Dempsey, P., & Hartley, D. (2001). *Efforts to Address Mental Health Workforce Needs in Underserved Rural Areas.* University of Southern Maine, Institute for Health Policy, Maine Rural Health Research Center (Working Paper #23).

Brown, D. L., & Schafft, K. (2011). *Rural People and Communities.* Malden, MA: Polity Press.

Brown, D., & Swanson, L. (Eds.). (2003). *Challenges for Rural America in the Twenty-First Century.* University Park: Pennsylvania State University Press.

Carr, P. J., & Kefalas, M. J. (2009). *Hollowing Out the Middle: The Rural Brain Drain and What It Means for America.* Boston: Beacon Press.

Carter, R. (2010). *Within Our Reach: Ending the Mental Health Crisis.* Emmaus, PA: Rodale Books.

Castle, E. (Ed.). (1995). *The Changing American Countryside: Rural People and Places.* Lawrence: University Press of Kansas.

Census.gov/geo/tiger/glossry2.html.

Duncan, C. (1999). *Worlds Apart: Why Poverty Persists in Rural America.* New Haven, CT: Yale University Press.

Elder, G., & Conger, R. (Eds.). (2000). *Children of the Land: Adversity and Success in Rural America.* Chicago: University of Chicago Press.

Fitchen, J. (1991). *Endangered Spaces, Enduring Places.* Boulder, CO: Westview Press.

Flora, C.B., & Flora, J.L. (2008). *Rural Communities, Legacy and Change* (3rd ed.). Philadelphia, PA: Westview Press/Perseus Books.

Grantham, D. (February 1, 2017). National Association of County Behavioral Health and Developmental Disability Directors (NACBHDD). *The Challenge of Affordable Health Care: The ACA and Beyond.* Washington, DC.

Harrington, M. (1997). *The Other America.* New York: Scribner.

Hartley, D., Bird, D., Lambert, D., & Coffin, J. (November, 2002). *The Role of Community Mental Health Centers as Rural Safety Net Providers.* Portland: University of Southern Maine, Edmund S. Muskie School of Public Service, Maine Rural Health Research Center (Working Paper #30).

Kagan, R., & Schlosberg, S. (1989). *Families in Perpetual Crisis.* New York: W.W. Norton.

Mohatt, D. F. (2016). *Rural Mental Health: Challenges and Opportunities Caring for the Country.* Boulder, CO: Western Interstate Commission for Higher Education.

Ranier, J. P. (2010). The road much less travelled: Treating rural and isolated clients. *Journal of Clinical Psychology: In Session*, 66(5), 475–478.
Semuels, A. (June 2, 2016). The Greying of Rural America. *The Atlantic*.
A Short History of the Farm Bill. (2016). Arlington, VA: Farm Policy Facts. www.farmpolicyfacts.org.
Smalley, K. B., Warren, J., & Rainer, J. (Eds.). (2012). *Rural Mental Health: Issues, Policies, And Best Practices*. New York: Springer.
Smalley, K. B., Yancey, C. T., Warren, J. C., Naufel, K., Ryan, R., & Pugh, J. L. (2010). Rural mental health and psychological treatment: A review for practitioners. *Journal of Clinical Psychology: In Session*, 66(5), 479–489.
Wood, R. E. (2008). *Survival of Rural America: Small Victories and Bitter Harvests*. Lawrence: University Press of Kansas.

9 Types of Mental Health Practitioners and Their Scopes of Practice

There are many different types of mental health practitioners, each with their own scope of practice. This chapter explores each level in the mental health care system, their training level, and reasons for selection, and presents some ideas for future additions to the system as well as ways practitioners of different kinds can collaborate for the benefit of individuals and communities. They include psychiatrists; psychologists; psychiatric nurse practitioners; licensed mental health counselors; licensed marriage and family therapists; licensed social workers; mobile crisis teams; crisis/respite workers; art therapists; dance, drama, music, and other creative arts therapists; and peer advocates and other mental health professionals.

Who is a mental health practitioner? Are all therapists equal? In the United States, there are three-quarters of a million people who have some kind of state statutory regulations and recognition in the form of approved credentials. They are known by a variety of names sure to confuse even the most savvy among us. They are known as psychiatrists, psychologists, licensed clinical social workers, psychiatric nurse practitioners, marriage and family therapists, counselors, creative arts therapists (including art, music, movement, and drama), licensed mental health counselors, addiction counselors, and peer counselors. For quite a while now, the number of those practicing at the master's level have outnumbered the number of practicing psychologists—and long before that, the number of practicing psychiatrists. Unfortunately, only a small fraction of these practicing professionals works in rural areas. Some believe that the psychiatry and psychology fields are seeking to increase their patient numbers and indirectly, their incomes, by enlarging the list of existing diagnostic categories to include more and more people, and creating syndromes and disorders by grouping collections of symptoms together in order for treatment for these individuals to be insurance reimbursable.

These disciplines have been known to have turf wars in order to protect their sustainability. According to Cummings, many accuse psychiatrists and psychologists of changing and "improving" the *Diagnostic and Statistical Manual* (DSM-5 is the most recent edition, having been published in

May 2015), increasing the number of diagnoses in order to include more and more people, and some accuse these fields of grouping any collection of symptoms so that treatment for these newly discovered conditions will be insurance reimbursable. For example, when the American Psychiatric Association redefined attention deficit hyperactivity disorder (ADHD) several years ago, the number of people who fell under the new guidelines nearly quadrupled.

Primary care providers are by far the most popular first stop for rural residents seeking help with mental health issues. Rural areas have less than half as many physicians per capita as urban areas. More than one-third of rural residents live in a federally designated HPSA (health professional shortage area). We must broaden the terms of the loan repayment program in order to attract more mental health providers to rural areas. The terms should include more rural counties and more types of qualified professionals, especially in counties with high poverty rates. Some money from the Obama-era American Recovery and Reinvestment Act (ARRA) was used to increase the number of awards; however, that money was a one-time gift. According to the HRSA Data Warehouse, as of July 6, 2011, there were 3,729 mental health HPSAs in the nation, with 61% of them located in non-metropolitan areas. In order to meet the mental health needs of the population, they calculated that upwards of 4,771 mental health practitioners would be required. The National Health Services Corporation (NHSC), which operates under the auspices of HRSA, has fulfilled 54% of mental health service provider needs in these shortage areas. This shows impressive improvement from the year 2000, when the NHSC was filling only 6% of the mental health manpower shortage. In 2008, for example, the Health Resources and Services Administration (HRSA) reported that there were 3,059 HPSAs for behavioral health, with a total of 77 million people living in these areas. Sixty-six percent of the behavioral health HPSAs were in rural areas. That statistic is totally unacceptable in this day and age. Mental health care must be accessible to all. Period.

What Is "Scope of Practice"?

Scope of practice describes the range of procedures, actions, and processes that a licensed practitioner in the health care field is permitted to undertake under the auspices of their state license. For example, some types of mental health practitioners have the scope of practice to diagnose; others do not. Some types of practitioners can prescribe psychotropic medications, others cannot. Each category of licensed mental health professional has its own governing licensing body, laws, and regulations defining the requirements for education, training, and the allowable practices under the type of license granted.

According to the Muskie School of Public Service at the University of Southern Maine, within the framework of state scope of practice laws, both public and private insurers have adopted a variety of payment policies for services provided by different types of mental health professionals. For example, Medicare does not recognize marriage and family therapists or professional counselors, but does recognize licensed clinical social workers, PhD psychologists, psychiatrists, and psychiatric nurse practitioners. Because commercial insurers such as Blue Cross and Blue Shield often follow the lead of Medicare, the result gives some master's level practitioners little incentive to practice in rural areas, even if they are willing. A practitioner who is unable to bill third party payers directly is not even considered qualified to work in a mental health clinic, depending on the state, and has to work under the auspices of a reimbursable provider. Both scenarios are met more easily in populated areas. In the absence of mental health workers who are eligible for insurance reimbursement, many rural residents receive mental health services from their primary care practitioners, who may consider themselves unqualified to provide such services and lack the time as well. While reimbursement policies may have greater effect than licensure laws in determining what kinds of professionals choose to practice in rural areas, some third party payers, such as Medicare, look to licensure laws as an indicator of which provider types they will allow to bill them directly. Historically, professional counselors have reacted against some of the other mental health professions, viewing them as disease-oriented, and have preferred to emphasize mental wellness. Without an agency to offer a salary or another professional under whose authority a rural practitioner can provide reimbursable services, barriers to direct reimbursement are also barriers to rural mental health practice.

The Muskie study concluded that for all of the mental health professions studies, little differentiation was found among the three primary mental health services. In other words, if a professional is allowed to perform one function, they are typically allowed to perform the others as well. Little variation was found from one state to another in the scope of practice for each credential. Considerable evidence was found that scope of practice laws should not be used as a basis for payment policies. Because diagnosis and psychotherapy are the only Medicare reimbursable mental health services of those studied here, one might expect to find the psychologists and social workers currently eligible for Medicare reimbursement to be licensed in these areas in all states. However, while no states specifically restrict them, some ignore and don't address them at all. Many states fail to mention psychotherapy in their scope of practice and many fail to mention diagnosis.

In addition, the study found evidence of a guild environment or turf wars in the field between practitioner categories. It also concluded that for the most part, state licensing laws fail to make specific regulatory accommodations for rural mental health practitioners.

The team that completed the study stated that they understand the frustration of policy makers when attempting to assess the adequacy of the mental health workforce to meet current needs. While there appears to be overlap in scope of services among the various professions, and some substitutability of one profession for another for some services, the language, training requirements, supervision requirements, and clinical approaches of the professions vary and are confusing.

As in New Hampshire, where licensees are required to obtain 25 hours of collaboration with other mental health professionals per renewal year, in Utah the Mental Health Professional Practice Act places professionals on an equal playing field in terms of the scope of their practices. Also, states vary on their requirements for the percentage of supervision time that can be done over the phone or by telephone or teleconferencing methods such as Skype, and their rules about who can supervise are confusing. Sometimes it has to be someone with the same credentialing, and other times it just needs to be a licensed professional. The latter is very helpful in rural areas, where it can help ease the shortage of practitioners.

The Muskie School of Public Service report on state laws and the mental health professions recommended that states simplify licensure and clarify clinical roles by combining regulatory functions for several professions into a single office or agency. A first step toward this end is either combining marriage and family therapy and licensed professional counseling into a single board, or creating a mental health professional practice act as Utah has done that addresses all mental health professions.

Another recommendation from the study is that state licensure laws do not support payers who choose not to reimburse marriage and family therapists or licensed professional counselors for essential mental health services. For example, the number of states permitting social workers to perform diagnosis and psychotherapy is not significantly different from the number permitting marriage and family therapists to perform those services. Yet Medicare chooses to reimburse social workers but not marriage and family therapists. Therefore, Medicare needs to reconsider its payment policies regarding non-physician mental health practitioners. States that have not already done so should consider vendorship laws to bring reimbursement policies into congruency with licensure laws by affirming the right of these professions to practice independently and be reimbursed by third party payers. An interim policy that might address rural needs would be to authorize direct reimbursement to these professions only in designated practitioner shortage areas.

Another potential solution brought forth by the Muskie study is that new strategies could be employed to reduce professional competition over the right to practice and be reimbursed. New Hampshire has addressed this issue by allowing candidates for licensure to be supervised by almost any mental health profession, and by requiring providers to provide proof that they do not work in professional isolation by submitting evidence of participation in a minimum of 25 hours of specified collaborative activities with members of other professions. Several other states have begun to address this issue through combined boards or mental health professional practice acts. The professional associations that represent these professions must provide stronger advocacy by taking the lead at the state level in working toward mental health professional practice acts and consolidated regulatory functions. New graduates of programs that train mental health professionals can begin to address rural needs soon after graduation, if arrangements can be made for them to receive supervision as required by most states for most professions. Supervision in rural areas may be easier to arrange in states where it is permissible to be supervised by a member of another profession. Another way of facilitating supervision is to explicitly allow telephone and telehealth technologies to be employed in supervision. A few states, such as Idaho, Wyoming, and Colorado, explicitly allow electronic supervision, acknowledging its necessity for rural practice sites. In rural states where electronic supervision is not permitted, professional associations, state rural health associations, offices of rural health, and Medicaid programs should work together to effect changes in licensure laws to allow it.

Psychiatrists

Psychiatrists are medical doctors who have continued their education to include expertise in psychiatric issues, treatments, and methods of practice. They can practice psychotherapy and prescribe psychotropic medication. They have studied for 4 years at the undergraduate level, another 4 years in medical school, and an additional 1–2 years in psychiatry.

Psychologists

Psychologists require a doctorate in psychology and generally need 2 years of supervised clinical experience in order to become licensed. They are expected to write an acceptable dissertation as a "gift" of research to the field. They cannot prescribe psychotropic medication except in New Mexico, Louisiana, Illinois, and Iowa (also considered by Arizona, Hawaii, Montana, Oregon, New Jersey, and Tennessee), but they can practice psychotherapy. Some states license psychologists at the master's level, but few allow them to practice independently.

When psychologists are able to prescribe psychotropic medications for clients (and unprescribe, which is also a complex procedure), patients are able to work with one health care provider for psychotherapy and medication management, if needed. Currently, most medications to treat mental disorders are prescribed by primary care physicians. However, they have not received extensive training in the diagnosis and treatment of mental health disorders, whereas psychologists do have that very specific in-depth knowledge.

In the states where it has become legal for psychologists to prescribe, they require additional training before they can begin. Psychologists who prescribe are able to ensure that all patients receive the proper combination of therapy and medication. Simply put, a prescribing psychologist offers integrated and comprehensive approach to care that can save time and money.

All licensed psychologists are highly trained, health care professionals holding a doctorate (PhD or PsyD) and extensive training in the diagnosis and management of mental illness. Graduate school for psychologists takes an average of 7 years, with coursework that includes the biological basis for human behavior.

After receiving a doctorate, a psychologist must complete between 1,500 and 6,000 hours of supervised clinical practice and take a national examination in order to become licensed (rules vary by state). In some states, an exam is also required. While each state develops its own educational requirements, the training for a licensed psychologist to prescribe is rigorous in all the proposed legislation. In Louisiana, psychologists must complete a post-doctoral master's degree in clinical psychopharmacology. New Mexico requires a minimum of 450 hours of additional instruction along with a 400-hour supervised practicum as part of its eligibility criteria. Illinois, psychologists seeking prescriptive authority must complete advanced, specialized training in psychopharmacology as well as a full-time practicum of 14 months of supervised clinical rotations in various settings such as hospitals, community mental health clinics, and correctional facilities. Psychologists must pass a certified exam in psychopharmacology. After completing their formal training, psychologists must coordinate care with a patient's primary care physician. Psychologists are also trained to know when to refer patients for the evaluation of other health problems. When all the training—doctoral and post-doctoral—is completed, prescribing psychologists have more training in diagnosing, treating, and prescribing for mental health disorders than primary care physicians. The need is great and the evidence is clear: allowing prescribing rights for psychologists is an essential step to providing thousands of patients with access to the medication portion of mental health care, especially in rural areas where shortages of practitioners are widespread.

Psychiatric Nurse Practitioners

Also called a mental health nurse practitioner, a psychiatric nurse practitioner (PNP) does many of the same things a psychiatrist does, including diagnosing mental illness and prescribing medication. Psychiatric nurse practitioners can also act as therapists, helping patients with depression, anxiety, suicidal ideations, and other conditions that can be remedied with counseling.

Their roles differ from psychologists or even psychiatrists and social workers, although all of the professionals in these positions can be involved in psychotherapy, but only advanced practice registered nurses (PNPs) and psychiatrists can prescribe medication. What may be more important is that all of these providers can practice independently, providing care where it may otherwise be inaccessible, although they are always under the authority of state law when it comes to scope of practice.

There are several pathways to becoming a psychiatric nurse practitioner, but no matter the path, the terminal degree is either a master of science in nursing (MSN) degree or a doctor of nursing practice (DNP) degree. An associate's degree in nursing (ADN) and experience working as a registered nurse (RN) are common admissions requirements for such programs. The time and commitment to complete coursework in a graduate-level program is considerable, but PNPs are very much in demand. For the psychiatric-mental health field, credentialing is offered through the American Nurses Credentialing Center (ANCC).

Licensed Mental Health Counselors or Licensed Marriage and Family Therapists

In order to become a licensed mental health counselor or licensed marriage and family therapists require a master's degree in counseling or psychology, performance of a 2,000–3,000-hour internship, and sometimes a qualifying examination. A portion of the internship is typically done during the graduate program and continued afterward.

Historically, one of the central philosophies of professional counseling has been that, unlike other disciplines in the mental health field, the focus has been on wellness and positive developmental health, not on psychopathology. The "developmental perspective" of professional counseling means that for the most part, mental health problems are viewed as normal responses to adverse life experiences. However, in their quest to be considered as equals in the world of third party insurance reimbursement, many have added training in pathology for that purpose. According to the American Counseling Association, the definition of professional counseling practice is the application of mental health, psychological, or human development principles through cognitive, affective, behavioral, or systemic intervention strategies that address wellness, personal growth, or career development, as well as pathology.

There is extreme lack of uniformity between states regarding the training, supervised experience, and examinations for professional counselors. Through licensing legislation, states have given a broad range of titles to those in the counseling profession. Some estimates say there are as many as 16 different titles used in counseling licensure laws throughout the country. The most common are professional counselor, mental health counselor, clinical counselor, and therapist.

Medicaid, the largest payer of mental health claims in the United States, has left many of its structural decisions to the states. As we know, in many states Medicaid does not cover certain types of licensed, credentialed professionals such as creative arts therapists, licensed mental health counselors, and others. There needs to be a uniform listing of the types of professionals Medicaid recipients are able to work with, as well as inclusion of these other types of mental health professionals, particularly in designated provider shortage areas. Perhaps there would be no shortage if this were accomplished. High poverty areas should be high priority, no question.

Marriage and family therapists are master's level practitioners who take a systemic, holistic approach regarding environments and relationships that affect the emotional well-being of the client. They are most similar to professional counselors, and are also not reimbursable by Medicare or Medicaid, a ruling that needs to change.

Licensed Clinical Social Workers

Licensed clinical social workers (LCSWs) require a master's degree in social work and 2 years of supervised clinical experience. Licensure is granted only after passing an examination. Social work is a blend of professional activities in the areas of poverty, social care, and acute mental health treatment. Social work practice is usually based on a medical model that includes diagnosis, treatment, and the notion of recovery or cure as an outcome. There are myriad ways in which a licensed clinical social worker can service their clients and impact people on societal, individual, and family levels. The most common career path is one of mental health counseling. With the help of an LCSW, clients can gain tremendous insight into their emotional makeup and find healing around past traumas. A social worker specializing in marriage and family might aid a family in working through their issues, facilitating dialogues, and ensuring that everyone's needs are met. This can result in marriages being strengthened that might otherwise end in divorce. The school counseling variation of the LCSW can help students be properly assessed so their unique needs are met, which in turn allows them to flourish within an academic setting.

The licensed clinical social worker can help families in many different ways. They can help to create child safety plans to keep children within the household. A school social worker might provide the missing insight so that a child might finally blossom at school, relieving stress in the family. With the help of the LCSW, the child can begin to express their needs in a healthy way and receive the attention they need to succeed academically. A social worker specializing in marriage and family counseling can help couples resolve their grievances and find a second chance for their relationship. In mental health counseling, a licensed clinical social worker can have a huge impact on an individual. During the course of treatment, a client can begin to understand, resolve, and heal from incredible traumas they have experienced during their lives, learn emotional literacy and coping skills, change their thinking patterns, and grow into their potential.

The education requirements to become a clinical social worker include a bachelor's degree in a closely related field, such as psychology, child development, social work, or sociology, and a master's degree in social work (MSW). Some states will then require you to accumulate supervised clinical experience. Finally, one must take their social work licensure exam. A MSW can earn additional "letters" in credentialing, such as an R (registered) or a C (certified) after working in the field under supervision for predetermined lengths of time.

Mobile Crisis Teams and Crisis Respite

Mobile crisis teams are made up of specially trained mental health professionals that respond to mental health crisis calls, bringing behavioral health care and criminal justice knowledge with them. The Mobile Crisis workers seek to de-escalate a crisis situation in order to prevent possible harm. They are usually funded enough to include a special car or vehicle and can therefore go to a client's home and work with them there. In remote rural areas this is no small feat: many have to travel an hour or more to the crisis call. However, this type of service is not widespread and needs to be. Use of mobile crisis units can result in alternatives to police or sheriff dispatches, detention, arrest, and hospital emergency room visits, can minimize the use of force, and can reduce trauma to the individual in crisis and a more positive start to treatment.

Crisis respite services provide safe places for people in crisis to be while they get the interventions they need to stabilize. With the closing of so many psychiatric hospitals around the country, they are often the only choice—if they are even available—for a person in crisis to remain safe while stabilizing. Waiting for a psychiatric hospital bed can take a quite a bit of time, and a person in crisis doesn't have that time to wait. At a crisis respite home, a person in crisis receives around-the-clock support from clinicians and peers to help those at risk until other services have room for them.

An increasing number of mobile crisis teams have vans that contain a small waiting area and a closed-off office space, and they travel to easily accessible sites in rural areas to have therapy appointments with people or to be available for a crisis. Although they can be expensive, such vans can be invaluable in providing services in rural and frontier areas. Some obstacles that would need to be overcome would be mastering the technology involved, the high cost of the vehicles, a lack of appropriate reimbursement from managed care, and whether or not cell phone service and internet service is available in the area for everyone's safety.

These are cost-effective interventions that need to have significant funding increases in order to meet the current need in our country.

Art Therapists, Music, Dance/Movement, and Drama Therapy

The creative arts therapies are advancing rapidly from being cutting edge treatment methods to settling down in the mainstream. They are evidence based and highly effective modalities for those willing to engage in them. The art product provides a third party in the therapeutic relationship that can be used for deflection and for self-expression when words are too difficult or emotional confusion reigns. It is a non-verbal way of working through issues within a therapeutic setting. Art therapy allows the client to depict a creative work symbolizing their inner world. The guiding premise in art therapy is that the product is not as important as the process of creating the artwork, and that there is healing inherent in the creative process. It's not about being good at it, it's about self-expression. Art therapy is used for assessment and diagnostic purposes.

The American Art Therapy Association (AATA) is a not-for-profit, professional, and educational organization dedicated to the growth and development of the art therapy profession. According to AATA, art therapy is an integrative mental health and human services profession that enriches the lives of individuals, families, and communities through active art-making, creative process, applied theory, and human experience within a psychotherapeutic relationship. Art therapy, facilitated by a professional art therapist, effectively supports personal and relational treatment goals as well as community concerns. Art therapy is used to improve cognitive and sensory motor functions, foster self-esteem and self-awareness, cultivate emotional resilience, promote insight, enhance social skills, reduce and resolve conflicts and distress, and advance societal and ecological change. Art therapists are master level clinicians who work with people of all ages across a broad spectrum of practice. Guided by ethical standards and scope of practice, their education and supervised training prepares them for culturally proficient work with diverse populations in a variety of settings. Honoring individuals' values and beliefs, art therapists work with people who are challenged with medical and mental health problems, as well as individuals seeking emotional, creative, and spiritual growth. Through integrative methods, art therapy engages the mind, body, and spirit in ways that are distinct from verbal articulation alone. Kinesthetic, sensory, perceptual, and symbolic opportunities invite alternative modes of receptive and expressive communication, which can circumvent the limitations of language. Visual and symbolic expression gives voice to experience and empowers individual, communal, and societal transformation.

Art therapists work with individuals, couples, families, and groups in diverse settings. Some examples include hospitals, schools, veterans' clinics, private practice, psychiatric and rehabilitation facilities, community clinics, crisis centers, forensic institutions, senior communities, and civic communities. Because of the intrinsic use of art by the client, art therapy can circumvent language barriers.

According to the AATA, through integrative methods art therapy engages the mind, body, and spirit in ways that are distinct from verbal articulation alone. In both trauma and addiction, the prefrontal cortex is "off-line" during activated emotional states, making therapies that do not use the prefrontal cortex such as cognitive therapies perfect in ways that cause lasting change for these conditions. Art therapy is also highly effective in working with a wide variety of populations such as autistic individuals, young children, adolescents, adults of any age including those with dementia, foster children, and is used in grief counseling, palliative care, medical care, and trauma cases.

Inaccurate use of art therapy often occurs due to a lack of in-depth knowledge about the profession. Another context in which art therapy may be inaccurately categorized includes professional trainings that furnish a certificate upon completion, which may mislead the participant into believing that he or she can practice art therapy. These sorts of trainings, workshops, and the like give attendees the erroneous impression that art therapy is a modality rather than a profession. Several products on the market may inaccurately identify the term "art therapy." Two such examples include art therapy apps and art therapy coloring books.

While the AATA does not discourage the use of art groups or coloring books for recreation and self-care, art activities must be distinguished from art therapy services provided by a credentialed art therapist. For more information, go to www.arttherapy.org.

Peer Advocates and Other Paraprofessionals

Many national organizations in the mental health field believe that of all the community-based tools in our system, peer supports (sometimes called

114   Types of Mental Health Practitioners

behavioral health aides) are among the most promising. By sharing their own personal experiences and lessons learned, they have been proven to help reduce incarceration and recidivism, and can intervene at any point in the process, from arrest through re-entering the community. Peer advocates are important for helping motivate people to make goals, get help, and empower themselves. Ron Manderscheid says:

> The Affordable Care Act already has increased private health insurance enrollment by about 11.7 million through the state Health Insurance marketplaces, and by about 6 million more through the state Medicaid Expansions. Of the former about a quarter of the enrollees have a behavioral health condition; among the latter, fully 40%. This translates into more than 5 million potential new consumers for a behavioral health care system that already is laboring to meet the needs of current participants. Thus, peer support services are an exceptionally welcome new resource—in my words, priceless!

Yet today, only 27 states fund peer support services as part of their state Medicaid plans.

Research shows that peer recovery support can result in reduced use of inpatient facilities, decreased costs to the mental health system, increased social functioning, empowerment, community engagement, and engagement in treatment.

There are various models of peer advocates emerging. Some focus more on acting as care coordinators or case managers, others focus on the use of mental health first aid by trained lay people. One thing is true across the board regarding peer advocates: all models are cost-effective and help provide deeply needed services in sorely underserved areas. All models are being adapted and improved on. Research dollars are needed in order to quantify what we believe to sound, cost-effective practice as evidence based. Many peer advocate programs lack a stable source of funding.

Several national agencies are undertaking efforts to promote this cost-effective type of provider. Mental Health America has proposed a peer training certification called the National Certified Peer Specialist. The Substance Abuse and Mental Health Services Administration (SAMHSA) has identified and developed a set of core competencies for peer workers in mental health settings. The National Alliance on Mental Illness (NAMI) has a program called Credentialed Family Peer Advocates. These volunteers are trained to empower and support individuals who have utilized mental health services in the past or present. The purpose of the program is to provide mutual support to those who just need someone to talk to, someone who understands what they are experiencing. All services are free of charge, are person centered and individualized. For more information, or to apply, visit the website of Families Together in New York State (www.ftnys.org).

Some drawbacks of the peer advocate or behavioral health aide role could include inadequacies in case documentation and organizational skills, managing job related stress, skills to develop appropriate prevention programs, clinical assessment skills, and the ability to handle the dynamics of client grief and loss. Because they are not licensed mental health professionals, their training needs to cover a wide range of topics including, but not limited to assessment and evaluation, establishing a helping relationship, treatment planning and implementation, referral sources, service coordination, client and family education, documentation, ethics, treatment and recovery models, and clinical supervision (NACBHDD).

Despite the proven value of peer supports, just 37 of 50 state Medicaid plans reimburse for peer support services. It will take a great deal of advocacy in order to get support through every state (NACBHDD).

A Peer Services Toolkit is available online at www.acmha.org.

Pastoral Counselors

For people who are more comfortable in a religious context, pastoral counselors fill a void in the mental health field. Pastoral counseling is a branch of counseling in which psychologically trained ministers, rabbis, priests, and other trained clergy provide therapy services. Pastoral counselors often integrate modern psychological thought and method with traditional religious training in an effort to address psychospiritual issues in addition to the traditional spectrum of counseling services. Pastoral counselors are representatives of the faith, beliefs, and traditions of their chosen religion and are affirmed by their religious communities. Pastoral counseling offers a relationship to that understanding of life and faith and can help with mental health issues. Pastoral counseling uses both psychological and theological resources to help people grow into their full potential, to overcome trauma, prevent suicide, grieve in a healthy way, and overcome addictions, because spirituality is an important part of recovery for many.

Primary Care Physicians (PCPs)—Issues With Providing Psychotropic Medications

Research has shown that rural residents are more likely to use their primary care physician versus psychotherapy for treatment of mental health disorders compared to urban residents. This is due to the likelihood that rural residents are amenable to receiving treatment for a mental illness from their primary care physician, making it more likely that they are more likely to use pharmacology rather than psychotherapy for treatment of mental health issues than their urban counterparts. For obvious reasons, many PCPs are uncomfortable prescribing and overseeing psychotropic medicine to patients.

Itinerant Counseling/Outreach

Itinerant counseling can be done by any of the aforementioned qualified mental health professionals. It can include visiting the client/family in the home and seeing how they interact in their own environment and the interpersonal dynamics, or in school settings that could show how a child interacts with peers and in structured setting with many expectations. Either of these settings contributes to a client's increased sense of authentication and validation.

There are a few drawbacks and potential problems with this model of care. One potential drawback is the lack of insurance reimbursement. Travel can be difficult in inclement weather, and many rural roads are not paved. Cell phone service is critical for itinerant counselors to have access to cell phone service for safety reasons, and many rural areas are not up to speed with coverage. Rural counselors need to understand and be able to work with not only the emotional issues, values, and characteristics in the rural culture, but the physical makeup of rurality as well. For example, I once followed a client to her barn where she milked a cow while we continued our conversation. I keep mud boots in my trunk for just such occasions, and it was valuable to me as a clinician to watch her at work in her own surroundings. In another family I was expected to be comfortable meeting with the family in their kitchen, with steaming mugs of coffee at their long farm table. I have found that families who voluntarily seek this method of counseling are warm and welcoming, and much quicker to engage with me.

More research on this model of service in rural areas needs to be done, but I believe it will be found to be a highly effective, cost-efficient tool in a great many rural cases.

Training for Rural Work

Training for mental health professionals should automatically include at minimum some familiarity with rural issues, and at present very few programs do. In my own graduate education there was no specific exposure to working with rural populations, even though I consider my education to be top rate. It has been suggested that clinicians should be exposed to and have specific training in areas such as things particular to a generalist practice, administration and management of a clinic or mental health office, collaboration and networking, research skills, personal and community values, consultation skills, supervision skills, technological advances such as telepsychology, rural issues, politics, culture, additional prevention training, program development and evaluation, grant writing, and rural ethics issues. Although rural practitioners need to be generalists, they need to have more than one course in alcohol and drug abuse in order to help combat the current drug epidemic. They should be aware that if they choose to work in a rural area, they need to be prepared to face professional issues such as isolation, lack of continuing education opportunities (although this is changing due to webinars), government regulations and restrictions, understanding of rural culture, lack of appropriate and sufficient numbers of referral sources, and lack of adequate agency resources. No one wants to accept a job in a rural area only to find out they are miserable living in a rural environment. Being educated about these issues in advance can turn a rural professional experience into a wonderful and lasting one.

References

Bain, S. F. (November, 2010). Itinerant counseling services for rural communities: A win/win opportunity. *Journal of Rural Community Psychology*, E13(1).

Berg-Cross, L., Reviere, R., Miller, J., Chappell, A., & Salmon, A. (2001). Certification of mental health advocates: A call to action. *Journal of Rural Community Psychology*, E14(1).

Bird, D.C., Dempsey, P., & Hartley, D. (2001). *Efforts to Address Mental Health Workforce Needs in Underserved Rural Areas.* University of Southern Maine, Institute for Health Policy, Maine Rural Health Research Center (Working Paper #23).

Brown, D., & Swanson, L. (Eds.). (2004). *Challenges for Rural America in the Twenty-First Century.* University Park: Pennsylvania State University Press.

Carter, R. (2010). *Within Our Reach: Ending the Mental Health Crisis.* Emmaus, PA: Rodale Books.

Cornell University. (2010). *Poverty, Local and Regional Government, Energy, Economic and Workforce Development, Agriculture and Food Systems.* Ithaca, NY. www.cornell.edu.

Florence, J.A., Goodrow, B., Wachs, J., Grover, S., & Olive, K.E. (2007). Rural health professions education at East Tennessee State University: Survey of graduates from the first decade of the community partnership program. *Journal of Rural Health*, Winter, 23(1), 77–83.

Ginsberg, L.H. (2005). Social *Work in Rural Communities* (4th ed.). Alexandria, VA: Council on Social Work Education.

Gladding, S.T. (1997). *Community and Agency Counseling.* Upper Saddle River, NJ: Prentice-Hall.

Goldman, H.H., Buck, J.A., & Thompson, K.S. (2009). *Transforming Mental Health Services: Implementing the Federal Agenda for Change.* Arlington, VA: American Psychiatric Association.

Grantham, D. (July 1, 2016). National Association of County Behavioral Health and Developmental Disability Directors (NACBHDD). *Under the Microscope: A Single National Standard for Peer Specialist Certification.* Washington, DC.

Hartley. D., Bird, D., Lambert, D., & Coffin, J. (November, 2002). *The Role of Community Mental Health Centers as Rural Safety Net Providers.* Portland: University of Southern Maine, Edmund S. Muskie School of Public Service, Maine Rural Health Research Center (Working Paper #30).

Hartley, D., Ziller, E., Lambert, D., Loux, S., & Bird, D. (2002, October). *State Licensure Laws and the Mental Health Professions: Implications for the Rural Mental Health Workforce.* Portland: University of Southern Maine, Edmund S. Muskie School of Public Service, Maine Rural Health Research Center (Working Paper #29).

Imig, A. (July 12, 2016). *Small But Mighty: Perspectives of Rural Mental Health Counselors.* The Professional Counselor. www.nbcc.org.

Jameson, J., & Blank, M. (2007). The role of clinical psychology in rural mental health services: Defining problems and developing solutions. *Clinical Psychology: Science and Practice*, 14, 283–298.

Junge, M. B. (2010). *A Modern History of Art Therapy in the United States*. Springfield, IL: Charles C. Thomas.

Kennedy Forum. (2016). *Navigating the New Frontier of Mental Health and Addiction: A Guide for the 115th Congress*. www.parityregistry.org; www.thekennedyforum.org; www.paritytrack.org.

Kennedy, J. F. (October 31, 1963). *Remarks on Signing Mental Retardation Facilities and Community Health Centers Construction Bill (Speech)*. Signing S. 1576, the Community Mental Health Act of 1963. White House Cabinet Room, Washington, DC: John F. Kennedy Presidential Library and Museum. JFKPOF-047-045.

Kennedy, P. J. (2015). *A Common Struggle: A Personal Journey Through the Past and Future of Mental Illness and Addiction*. New York: Blue Rider Press.

Kos, M. E., & DeStefano, T. J. (2000). The investigation of the developmental course of burnout among rural clinicians. *Journal of Rural Community Psychology*, E14(1).

Layard, R., & Clark, D. M. (2015). *Thrive: How Better Mental Health Care Transforms Lives and Saves Money*. Princeton, NJ: Princeton University Press.

Manderscheid, R. (August 28, 2016). Last Chance to Pass Mental Health Reform? *Behavioral Healthcare Magazine*. www.behavioral.net.

Meyer, D., Hamel-Lambert, J., Tice, C., Safran, S., Bolon, D., Rose-Grippa, K. (2005). Recruiting and retaining mental health professionals to rural communities: An interdisciplinary course in Appalachia. *Journal of Rural Health*, Winter, 21(1), 89–91.

Mohatt, D. F. (2016). *Rural Mental Health: Challenges and Opportunities Caring for the Country*. Boulder, CO: Western Interstate Commission for Higher Education.

Morris, J. (2009). Marriage and family therapists expand access to mental health services in rural areas. *Journal of Rural Community Psychology*, Summer, E12(1).

National Association of Rural Mental Health. www.NARMH.org.

National Rural Health Association, Government Affairs Office (NRHAGAO). (October, 2008). *Policy Position: Workforce Series—Rural Behavioral Health*. Washington, DC.

New Freedom Commission on Mental Health. (2003). *Achieving the Promise: Transforming Mental Health Care in America*. Final. DHHS Pub. Co. SMA-03-3832. Rockville, MD.

Olfman, S. (2015). *The Science and Pseudoscience of Children's Mental Health*. Santa Barbara, CA: Praeger.

Rainer, J. P. (2010). The road much less traveled: Treating rural and isolated clients. *Journal of Clinical Psychology: In Session*, 66(5), 475–478.

Robert, D. (Ed.). (1992). *Psychological Practice in Small Towns and Rural Areas*. Binghamton, NY: Haworth Press.

Rural Policy Research Institute. (2016). www.rupri.org.

Smalley, K. B., Warren, J., & Rainer, J. (Eds.). (2012). *Rural Mental Health: Issues, Policies, and Best Practices*. New York: Springer.

Smalley, K. B., Yancey, C. T., Warren, J. C., Naufel, K., Ryan, R., & Pugh, J. L. (2010). Rural mental health and psychological treatment: A review for practitioners. *Journal of Clinical Psychology: In Session*, 66(5), 479–489.

Smith, A. (2003). Rural mental health counseling: One example of practicing whatever the research preaches. *Journal of Rural Community Psychology*, E6(2), Fall.

Stamm, B. H. (Ed.). (2003). *Rural Behavioral Health Care*. Washington, DC: American Psychological Association.

Townsend, W. (2010). Recovery services in rural settings, strengths and challenges influencing behavioral healthcare service delivery. *Rural Mental Health*, 34(1), 23–32.

US Department of Health and Human Services. (1999). Rockville, MD: Substance Abuse and Mental Health Services Administration. Promising Practices. Rockville, MD: Office of Rural Health Policy, Health Resources and Services Administration.

Van Hecke, S. (2012). *Behavioral Health Aides: A Promising Practice for Frontier Communities*. National Center for Frontier Communities and the Frontier and Rural Expert Panel.

Wilson, W., Bangs, A., & Hatting, T. (February, 2015). *The Future of Rural Behavioral Health*. National Rural Health Association Policy Brief. www.ruralhealthnet.org.

Ziller, E. (2002). *State Licensure Laws and the Mental Health Professions: Implications for the Rural Mental Health Workforce*. Portland, ME: Cutler Institute for Health and Social Policy.

10 Treatment Philosophies and Models

We are in the age of the cognitive revolution. However, has that become a one-size-fits-all way of thinking? There are several helpful evidence-based cognitive models that are powerful tools for clients, but is that all there is? This chapter surveys some little used theories that lend themselves beautifully to rural clientele. They include ecopsychology, the Sanctuary Model, community psychology, trauma-informed therapy, and the public health approach.

The Flavor of the Year: Beyond CBT for All

The big change since the start of the 21st century is that we are now in what many in the field call the cognitive revolution. It is characterized by a move toward evidence-based therapies, which are easier to quantify than the popular depth psychologies of the 19th and 20th centuries such as psychoanalytic and interpersonal therapies. Some practitioners believe that this over-quantification results in a rigid, inflexible therapy that lends itself to a one-size-fits-all methodology. Those practitioners who are not affiliated with the academic or science-based psychologies believe that clinical experience is equally important as research results. Then again, there are many who are comfortable in the middle area between the academic- or science-based and the clinical skills–based therapies. These evidence-based life-changing therapies are cost-effective to the health care system. The cost is mostly recouped in the reduced cost of physical health care for people who have physical as well as mental health problems. On top of that is the saving on welfare payments. So there would be no net cost increase in making these therapies more widely available.

In the 1980s the trend was for brief psychotherapies, and managed care companies were quick to embrace this trend for its cost-effectiveness, with limited number of sessions on a majority of health care plans. Unfortunately, these limitations are still in play, as cognitive behavioral therapy (CBT) usually involves between 12 and 20 sessions. It utilizes the strength of the therapeutic relationship, without which therapy is unsuccessful, and a treatment therapists must be trained in, the goal of which is to help the client to change his or her thought patterns.

Ecopsychology

Theodore Roszak, well-known author and scholar, coined the term ecopsychology (he also coined the phrase "counterculture"). Ecopsychology is the merging of ecological and psychological principles. The field seeks to develop ways of expanding the emotional connection between individuals and the natural world, thereby assisting individuals with developing sustainable lifestyles and remedying alienation from nature.

Many researchers propose that an individual's connection to nature can improve their interpersonal relationships and emotional well-being. An integral part of this practice is to remove psychotherapy, and the individual, from the interior of office buildings and homes and place them outdoors. According to the precepts of ecopsychology, a walk in the woods or a city park is refreshing because it is what humans evolved to do. Richard Louv's *Last Child in the Woods: Saving Our Children From Nature-Deficit Disorder* discusses in detail how the exposure of children to nature can assist in treating mental disorders, including attention deficit hyperactivity disorder (ADHD).

A central premise of ecopsychology is that while in modern times the human mind is affected and shaped by the modern social world, its deep structure is inevitably adapted to, and informed by, the more-than-human natural environment in which it evolved. According to biologist E.O. Wilson, human beings have an instinct to connect emotionally with nature.

The field of ecopsychology extends beyond the conventional realms of psychology, which traditionally considered the psyche to be a matter of relevance to humans alone. Ecopsychology examines why people continue environmentally damaging behavior, and seeks to develop methods of positive motivation for adopting sustainable practices. Evidence suggests that many environmentally damaging behaviors are addictive at some level, and thus are more effectively addressed through positive emotional fulfillment rather than by inflicting shame. Other names used to refer to ecopsychology include depth ecology, Gaia psychology, psycho-ecology, ecotherapy, environmental psychology, green psychology, transpersonal ecology, global therapy, green therapy, Earth-centered therapy, re-earthing, and nature-based psychotherapy.

Another premise of ecopsychology is that steps taken to accept and notice nature can sharpen the senses and help people cultivate new skills. For example, the ability to track and navigate through a wilderness is improved if nature is noticed and accepted rather than feared. Similarly, ecopsychology proposes that sailors who appreciate the sea gain a keen sense for breeze directions.

Ecopsychology explores how to develop emotional bonds with nature. When nature is explored and viewed without judgment, it gives the sensations of harmony, balance, timelessness, and stability. Ecopsychology largely rejects reductionist views of nature that focus upon rudimentary building blocks, such as genes, and that describe nature as selfish and a struggle to survive.

In its exploration of how to bond with nature, ecopsychology is interested in the examples provided by a wide variety of ancient and modern cultures that have histories of embracing nature. Examples include Aboriginal, pagan, Buddhist, and Hindu cultures as well as shamanism. Of interest is how identity becomes entwined with nature, so that loss of those sacred places is far more devastating to indigenous people than we have previously understood. Native American stories, in particular, illustrate a socially recognized sense of community between humans and the natural landscape. The Māori philosophy and practice of eco-guardianship and preservation emphasizes a deep connection between humans and their environment. Eastern Orthodox monks led a contemplative life deeply intertwined with nature. Other lessons include how to live sustainably within an environment and the self-sacrifices made to tolerate natural limits, such as population control or a nomadic existence that allows the environment to regenerate. Certain indigenous cultures have developed methods of psychotherapy involving the presence of trees, rivers, and astronomical bodies.

Ecopsychologists have begun detecting unspoken grief within individuals, an escalation of pain and despair, felt in response to widespread environmental destruction and climate change. Ecopsychologists believe that if a culture is disconnected from nature, then various aspects of human life will be negatively impacted. They also believe that without the influence of nature, humans are prone to a variety of delusions, and that to some degree life in the wild forms the basis for human sanity and optimal psychological development. The topic is explored in detail in Paul Shepard's book *Nature and Madness*. It is also proposed that separation from outdoor contact causes a loss of sensory and information-processing ability that was developed over the course of human evolution, which was spent in direct reciprocity with the environment. Although relatively new on the psychological radar, ecopsychology is a growing branch on the tree of psychological theory, especially given climate change and other serious ecological issues of our times.

The Sanctuary Model

Developed by Sandra Bloom, the goal of the Sanctuary Model is to help children who have experienced the damaging effects of interpersonal violence, abuse, and trauma. The model is intended for use by residential treatment settings for children, public schools, domestic violence shelters, homeless shelters, group homes, outpatient and community-based settings, juvenile justice programs, substance abuse programs, parenting support programs, acute care settings, and other programs aimed at assisting children.

Bloom indicates that the model's approach helps organizations create a truly collaborative and healing environment that improves efficacy in the treatment of traumatized individuals, reduces restraints and other coercive practices, builds cross-functional teams, and improves staff morale and retention.

Seeking Safety, as the program is called, is designed to be a therapy for trauma, post-traumatic stress disorder (PTSD), and substance abuse. The belief is that this model works for individuals or with groups; with men, women, or mixed-gender groups; and can be used in a variety of settings, such as outpatient, inpatient, and residential.

Bloom indicates that the key principles of Seeking Safety are safety as the overarching goal, integrated treatment, a focus on ideals to counteract the loss of ideals in both PTSD and substance abuse, knowledge of four content areas (cognitive, behavioral, interpersonal, and case management), and attention to clinical processes.

The Sanctuary Model came out of Bloom's 30 years of involvement in therapeutic settings, particularly her work from 1980 to 2001 in short-term, inpatient psychiatric settings for adults traumatized as children. In these settings the doors were not locked. No one was isolated or restrained, either physically or with chemicals to dull affect.

In 10 days of inpatient psychiatric treatment, people had a very different experience from their previous experiences. They were able to internalize an alternative philosophy that included respect and participation in a community. They learned that they were not sick, crazy, or bad, but rather injured, and as a result they had problems. They became part of a community based on shared responsibility that supported them in their efforts to stop doing the things that made them feel bad. Traditionally, they had merely been given a label and a diagnosis, but that didn't help them learn how to help themselves. Their systems of care were not trauma-informed. As they learned more about the effects of trauma, they showed people the effect their experiences had on their bodies and minds.

Bloom and her colleagues developed and taught clients how to use the S.E.L.F. tool (part of the Sanctuary Tool Kit), which represents four key aspects of recovery from bad experiences: Safety, Emotional Management, Loss, and Future.

Bloom writes that as the Sanctuary Model is implemented, tangible improvements are seen in morale, staff burnout decreases, as does worker's compensation applications and vicarious trauma (transferred from client to staff), as well as violence and the need for seclusions and restraint.

Community Psychology

There is a branch of psychology called community psychology, which focuses on an individual and his or her interactions within communities as well as the wider society. It began as a natural outgrowth of the Community Mental Health Movement. Community psychologists seek to understand the quality of life of individuals, communities, and society. The aim of community psychologists is to enhance quality of life through collaborative research and action. Community psychology employs various psychological perspectives to address issues of communities, the relationships within them, and people's attitudes and behavior toward themselves in their environment and in relationship to others in the community.

The early community psychologists embraced the concepts of collaboration, patient advocacy, networking, and team treatment. These concepts became the hallmark of rural practice and meshed nicely with a psychologist's training in the management of group dynamics, the development of behavioral paradigms, and the collection and interpretation of data. Rural psychologists began to integrate the principles of psychological science and practice with the little that was available in the way of grassroots agencies and resources. These included the clergy and religions institutions, social service agencies, law enforcement, courts, school districts, state mental health authorities, primary care physicians, and the community hospital. Community psychology asserted the importance of social and environmental factors in changing behavior, supported system-oriented interventions, and began to advocate for prevention and the treatment of targeted populations rather than just the alleviation of psychopathology. The community psychologist focused on the management of local community resources and caretakers and the psychological condition of the patient, and actively reached out to patients and groups to foster early identification and intervention. These psychologists adopted ecological approaches with flexible intervention styles and modalities as a vehicle to develop innovative programs. They tapped into whichever resources were available on the local level to solve psychological problems and to foster constructive social reform (Morris, pp. 4–5).

Trauma-Informed Therapy

While deserving a book of its own, trauma-informed therapy is a branch of psychology that is rapidly growing and shows no signs of slowing down in the foreseeable future. As we know, trauma has devastating effects on the mental, physical, social, and spiritual wellness of an individual. Volumes have been written on the subject in the last several decades, with more books pouring out of publishing houses every year.

While the nuts and bolts of therapy with traumatized individuals varies widely according to which psychological philosophy it is linked to, many use a blend of cognitive behavioral therapy (CBT), cognitive processing therapy, trauma-focused CBT, and a person-centered, strengths-based model of care. As the number of people globally who are traumatized increases exponentially with unprecedented killer storms, terrorism, political displacement, and those suffering from grief, disease, and droughts, trauma-informed therapy will become an even more important tool than it is already.

The Public Health Approach

The Center for Community-Based Children's Mental Health Research and Policy proposes a three-tiered public health approach to mental health, including:

- Universal: A model of mental health promotion at the universal level emphasizes leveraging community settings (schools, park districts,

community centers) to meet mental health needs. Inherent in most of these settings are opportunities to foster skills, develop relationships, and engage in healthy functioning. Empowering front-line workers and increasing organizational capability will enhance the ability for these settings to deliver the highest quality services.
- Targeted: These interventions prioritize care for high-risk groups. Children of parents with mental illness, families living in poverty, or individuals exhibiting early symptoms constitute this high-risk category. Targeted interventions can be integrated into primary care offices, emergency rooms, social service agencies, and schools.
- Intensive: Current rates of mental illness diagnoses in our country exceed the availability of mental health providers. In the same way, nutrition, exercise, and wellness programs can have an impact on diabetes, cardiovascular disease, and cancer. Providing the universal and targeted interventions can decrease the number of mental health disorders, individuals exhibiting symptoms, and more severe impairments.

Trying to restructure the current approaches by revising psychotherapy, no matter how innovatively, addresses a small part of the problem. It does not consider the poor. It does not look at the most vulnerable populations. It does not think of social determinants that can make communities more susceptible or make issues worse. Only a comprehensive and integrated public health model can address the pervasive societal problems and inequalities that underlie our country's mental health needs.

A public health approach to mental health has been advocated by the World Health Organization and provides the guiding framework for Every Moment Counts, which emphasizes the promotion of mental health and the prevention of and intervention for mental illness, thereby reducing stigma. Some leaders in the field of children's mental health have also promoted the adoption of a multi-tiered public health approach. This framework supports a change in thinking from the traditional, individually focused, deficit-driven model of mental health intervention to a whole-population, strength-based approach. This paradigm shift to addressing complex children's mental health calls for an accompanying shift in practices, to better prepare all school personnel (e.g., teachers, administrators, para-educators, and related service providers) to proactively address the mental health needs of all students and to burn the punitive model.

Within this public health model, a range of intervention services are provided and include:

Promotion: enhancing competencies; optimizing positive mental health
Prevention: reducing risks; minimizing mental health problems
Intensive, individualized interventions are provided to reduce the effects of a mental illness and restore mental health.

References

Beck, A. (1979). *Cognitive Therapy and the Emotional Disorders.* New York: Plume.

Bloom, S. (1997). *Creating Sanctuary: Toward the Evolution of Sane Societies.* New York: Routledge.

Carter, R. (2010). *Within Our Reach: Ending the Mental Health Crisis.* Emmaus, PA: Rodale Books.

Gladding, S. T. (1997). *Community and Agency Counseling.* Upper Saddle River, NJ: Council on Social Work Education.

Goleman, D. (2009). *Ecological Intelligence.* New York: Broadway Books.

Herman, J. (1997). *Trauma and Recovery: The Aftermath of Violence From Domestic Abuse to Political Terror.* New York: Basic Books.

Kennedy Forum. (2016). *Navigating the New Frontier of Mental Health and Addiction: A Guide for the 115th Congress.* www.parityregistry.org; www.thekennedyforum.org; www.paritytrack.org.

Kennedy, P. J. (2015). *A Common Struggle: A Personal Journey Through the Past and Future of Mental Illness and Addiction.* New York: Blue Rider Press.

Levine, P. (1997). *Waking the Tiger: Healing Trauma.* Berkeley, CA: North Atlantic Books.

Levine, P. (2010). *In an Unspoken Voice: How the Body Releases Trauma and Restores Goodness.* Berkeley, CA: North Atlantic Books.

Lightburn, A., & Sessions, P. (2006). *Handbook of Community-Based Clinical Practice.* New York: Oxford University Press.

Morris, J. A. (1997). *Practicing Psychology in Rural Settings.* Washington, DC: American Psychological Association.

Olfman, S. (2015). *The Science and Pseudoscience of Children's Mental Health.* Santa Barbara, CA: Praeger.

Roszak, T. (1995). *Ecopsychology: Restoring the Earth, Healing the Mind.* Oakland, CA: Sierra Club Books.

Smalley, K. B., Warren, J., & Rainer, J. (Eds.). (2012). *Rural Mental Health: Issues, Policies, and Best Practices.* New York: Springer.

Smalley, K. B., Yancey, C. T., Warren, J. C., Naufel, K., Ryan, R., & Pugh, J. L. (2010). Rural mental health and psychological treatment: A review for practitioners. *Journal of Clinical Psychology: In Session,* 66(5), 479–489.

Smith, A. (2003). Rural mental health counseling: One example of practicing what the research preaches. *Journal of Rural Community Psychology,* E6(2), Fall.

Taubenheim, A., & Tiano, J. (2012). Rationale and modifications for implementing parent-child interaction therapy with rural Appalachian parents. *Rural Mental Health,* Fall/Winter.

Van der Kolk, B. (2015). *The Body Keeps the Score: Brain, Mind and Body in the Healing of Trauma.* New York: Penguin.

Whitaker, R. (2010). *Anatomy of an Epidemic.* New York: Broadway Books.

11 Issues in Rural Practice

This chapter investigates ethics in rural mental health, which have many specific circumstances as compared with urban areas, which have their own unique situations. From boundary issues and confidentiality in the age of HIPAA, and from professional isolation to the need to be a generalist, rural mental health practitioners of all types need to learn how to blend in to their rural communities. Because there is a lack of anonymity, frequent gossip, and public scrutiny in small towns, practitioners need to know how to cope in order to thrive. If they can't thrive, they can't be of much help to their clients. There is little preparation in education programs for mental health practitioners for rural practice and rural life, and that needs to change.

Ethics in Rural Mental Health

Mental health ethical codes are often difficult to uphold in rural and small-town areas. Prevailing standards in training, ethical codes, and regulations are usually developed in urban areas and not easily applied in rural and small town practice, nor are they necessarily applicable. The extent to which lack of anonymity and considerable public investigation and knowledge about the practitioner's personal life often creates major difficulty in rendering professional services cannot be overemphasized. These issues are addressed in graduate school. It is difficult to be anonymous in small towns. Try going to the store to pick up milk and bread quickly. You run into all kinds of people, some of whom you have messages for, some of whom you haven't seen in a while, some who want to know how your mother-in-law is feeling since her recent hospitalization. There is rarely anything quick about it. And that's what small town community is about. Many rural residents are mistrustful of outsiders until they have proven themselves to be trustworthy, which takes years. Becoming fully accepted also takes showing up at community events, whether fairs or local town business or school board meetings.

It is of the utmost importance to set clinical relationship boundaries by addressing the possibility of chance encounters with clients early on in the first session. The solution can be very simple and straightforward. It is important that the client understand that this is directly related to the value being placed on confidentiality and protecting their privacy. Some people like to be acknowledged and would feel hurt if the clinician did not acknowledge them in a public place. My practice is to address this in the first session by letting the client know that I will acknowledge them in public by saying hello and continuing on if that meets with their approval. This way we can acknowledge each other, but given the small town phenomenon of people wearing multiple hats, no one needs to know how we know each other. I have found that mostly everyone agrees to this plan, and it has gone well when I have seen clients in public. I also make it clear, especially to children who are new to the idea of privacy, that they can tell others about our working together if they would like to, but I will not tell anyone else. Many children ask questions about which other children see me in my office, and they feel confused when I refuse to answer and explain the confidentiality factor. Once they understand, they usually relax and focus on themselves. As members of the community at large learn that the clinician is skilled at maintaining appropriate boundaries and confidentiality, they usually gain credibility and can even become more sought out, sometimes even for community-wide committees and boards that involve mental health, in addition to gaining clients. I have worked with families that were related by marriage without the other side being aware, with a trio of teenage girls who discovered one night on a sleepover that they were all working with me and had been for quite a while, and with my daughter's classmates. I deliberately do not have a shingle in front of my office for confidentiality reasons.

It is also important for clients to understand the boundaries of clinical conversations, that they should only occur in the privacy of the office. Clients also need to understand the circumstances under which confidentiality can be broken: if I as the clinician feel that the client is in danger of hurting themselves or others. And I make it clear that any action I would take would be to keep themselves and others safe.

Imig wrote in *The Professional Counselor* that to help close the geographic distance in rural areas, participants met with clients in a variety of non-traditional settings to lessen the physical gap. Settings included town libraries, churches, and schools. Not only does this help with the transportation issues inherent in rural areas, but it has the additional benefit of reducing stigma.

There is a relative lack of control that therapists working in small communities possess over what is known about them. The decline in anonymity that results from rural living is in direct correlation with an increase in multiple roles. As a result of these additional roles, the therapist will be considered by the patient as more of a multidimensional person. Likewise, the same phenomenon occurs by which the therapist appreciates the patient as multidimensional.

Rural practitioners also face the dilemma of hearing unsolicited information from people, and that information can be hard to filter. Sources for such information can be the local grapevine, community newsletters, the police blotter in the local newspaper, and people talking out of turn. I once saw three teenage girls, each on their own, with none knowing that the others were also working with me. At one point, they were purposely burning their hands with a salt solution as self-injurious behavior. I heard about it from one of the girls, then was made aware that the other two, who were never forthcoming about it, were also doing it to themselves. They figured out that they had me in common during a slumber party and were surprised.

Other Issues in Rural Mental Health

In *The Challenges of Rural Clinical Mental Health Counseling*, Daniel Weigel examined the multidisciplinary rural mental health literature base and found 17 prominent themes. They are the generalist nature of rural practice; personal and professional isolation in rural settings; extensive consultation and education services; lack of referral sources; collaboration with other agencies and professionals; geographic obstacles; lack of supervision and professional consultation opportunities; need for personal independence, creativity, flexibility; increased administrative and managerial responsibilities; use of indigenous resources and paraprofessionals; extensive advocacy services; lack of applied research in rural settings; heavy client caseloads; extensive preventative services; extensive crisis and on-call emergency tasks; lack of funding sources to provide needed services; and short-term service delivery demands.

I have often wondered how I have survived in a place such as this because it is so foreign from where I grew up in the outskirts of New York City. I think the answer is that rurality has seduced me by giving me what I have really needed, which is a sense of belonging and rootedness. It has also given me a sense of living closer to nature, which I thrive on. I am nurtured by living in this community, in this area with this flora and fauna and its human element.

Because it is a high poverty area, have to deal with some clients who can only pay very little, some who cannot pay at all, and some who cannot pay immediately.

There is a kind of inherent trust here, too, which I think is absent in most urban areas and that makes the job of the therapist easier and more likely to be successful. Of course, sometimes with certain people there is a huge initial sense of distrust, but many are open enough to allow that to change over time as they get to know me.

Keeping current educationally and clinically is more challenging in rural areas. Attending conferences for professional development and license maintenance is often geographically impossible. Although the formal part of my education ended years ago, I study, read, and research topics regularly in order to meet the challenge of helping those with special needs and situations. The side benefit of doing this is eliminating boredom for me, or, stated in the positive, providing myself with opportunities of learning new things. In my practice I am rarely bored or stale, partly owing to the nature of being a generalist and partly because of my personal intolerance for boredom and maintaining the status quo. My varied client list demands that I be creative, flexible, and aware of new research and theories. Some other commercial (for-profit) mental health clinics are very competitive. I believe they are acting in a totally inappropriate and unnecessary way. This is not a competitive "business" we are in. We ought to be supporting each other, referring to each other and collaborating when possible.

Eventually worry about being discovered fades to the background of a client's concern, as they realize that to be in therapy does not mean they are crazy. I don't view seeing clients in dual roles as an obstacle, but rather as a very workable and useful parameter to negotiate. Sometimes personal aspects of certain relationships need to be set aside for a period of weeks, months, or even years. The hope is that there is enough mutual trust between the individuals to know that there is mutual caring and respect.

In order to orient clients to be active participants in the therapy process, I have found it necessary to describe the responsibilities of therapist and those of the client and the therapeutic process itself right in the first session. I always emphasize that my office is a safe place, and children test that statement by using "bad" words, which meet with no consequence. They are typically shocked that they can get away with using such words. But it helps foster trust to bring more sensitive feelings into the conversation.

I once had a child tell me that he saw his daddy hitting his mommy and that mommy was bleeding. As a mandated reporter of such statements, I called the state hotline and explained the case to the woman on the other end of the phone. If the state deems it necessary, they will call the case in to my local Department of Social Services, who will make a visit to the home within hours. As she asked me questions, I it dawned on me that the parents of this child could easily figure out who made the call to "turn them in," or at least narrow it down to several people. I have a listed phone number, but even if I didn't, in this age of information, anyone can find out where I live, and I found this frightening. I felt I had put my family and myself in jeopardy. It reminded me of a time I was the only adult left in the building late in the afternoon, and a parent came in and proceeded to scream and threaten me. He was a parent I knew owned a gun, and who had a bad reputation for being hot-tempered. How could I know if he had his gun on him? My hand on the phone to call the police was all that stopped him before he stormed out, leaving me rattled and frightened.

Relationships in rural areas are not determined as much by intention or choice, as might be found in the city, but by proximity. In urban settings, in general, one does not of necessity socialize, have personal knowledge, or enjoy a personal relationship with those they interact with on a daily peripheral basis, nor is the city dweller likely to know the name of those who live on his or her block. In urban or suburban settings, one chooses relationships with a fair amount of intentionality—not merely because the person is present because the pool of available people to interact with is larger. In rural areas, the choices for relationships are more limited; everybody knows everybody, and interacts with most in very different ways. Sometimes we interact with the same person in multiple ways due to the phenomenon of wearing many hats. Life in the city is characterized by anonymity, whereas rural life is characterized by an unusual degree of openness: one's behavior and the behavior of one's family are not only open to public scrutiny, but become favorite topics of community discussion. It is akin to living in a glass house.

I have observed that movement between social classes is more fluid in rural settings. In the city, and definitely in suburbia, it is possible to avoid contact with blue collar workers. In rural areas, proximity to people crossing all class lines is common. In urban settings, relationships, particularly with professionals, are distant and formal. In a rural area, your doctor may be your best friend's mother. I have close friends who are old enough to be my mother, and others for whom I am old enough to be their mother. Age and social class factor in less than they would in urban or suburban areas when it comes to close relationships.

A sticky issue is that of bartering for professional services and general disapproval from ethics committees. However, I would argue that there are special circumstances that emerge in rural settings in which bartering is justifiable—and even desirable. I have done it on occasion. For example, I once accepted payment in the form of fresh vegetables from a farmer who couldn't afford to pay in money. It was a refreshing change of pace (the vegetables were delicious), and I would do it again if the situation presented itself. It is something that requires careful consideration and weight of the individual circumstances. One case was a woman who had no extra money after her monthly paycheck to pay me out of pocket. She had been a dog groomer before she retired, and so we placed a dollar value on each of our skills and she groomed my dog several times for me during the time we worked together. After very careful consideration, I decided that this was the only way she was going to be able to get treatment because the nearest Medicaid provider was over an hour away from her home. In the end it worked out well, but I never offer this option upfront, and have, in fact, turned people down in situations of bartering if they had another way of obtaining services. It is critical that clients feel the dignity of being able to pay for a service whether with cash or with a necessary service. Paying for therapy, whatever the cost, helps motivate a person to work harder.

The extent to which a lack of anonymity, gossip, and public scrutiny about a professional's personal life often makes providing services more complicated. If a practitioner's child gets in trouble with the law, or a partner is having an affair, very often everyone knows about it. And if they don't know the actual facts, they usually assume they do. It fits with the old expression, "If I heard it in the coffee shop down the street, it must be true."

Because most rural mental health practitioners have high caseloads and professional isolation in addition to the other stresses inherent in their jobs, they would do well to pay attention to their own self-care. Because of the nature of small towns, if they choose to engage in therapy themselves, they may need to seek a practitioner who is geographically distant. In order to prevent job burnout, practitioners need to be aware of knowing what nourishes them, and must be disciplined enough to make those things a regular part of their daily routines.

In order to help increase the workforce in rural areas, these issues need to be addressed in college and graduate programs so that prospective clinicians understand that these issues are complex but can be dealt with in satisfactory ways that can alleviate misunderstandings, and that this may be a small price to pay for a rural lifestyle that is well worth it. Professional organizations such as the American Psychological Association (APA) would do well to recognize the need for greater flexibility in leaving some things to the discretion of the professional in determining how to manage the delicate balance of working and living in small-town rural areas. These are unique situations that often require consideration on a case-by-case basis.

References

Addressing Mental Health Workforce Needs in Underserved Rural Areas: Accomplishments and Agriculture Is Vital to New York's Economy. (2015). Overland Park, KS: National Crop Insurance Services.

Bagalman, E. (2016). *The Helping Families in Mental Health Crisis Reform Act of 2016.* Washington, DC: Congressional Research Service.

Bailey, C., Jensen, L., & Ransom, E. (2014). *Rural America in a Globalizing World.* Morgantown: West Virginia University Press.

Berg-Cross, L., Reviere, R., Miller, J., Chappell, A., & Salmon, A. (2001). Certification of mental health advocates: A call to action. *Journal of Rural Community Psychology,* E14(1).

Bird, D.C., Dempsey, P., & Hartley, D. (2001). *Efforts to Address Mental Health Workforce Needs in Underserved Rural Areas.* University of Southern Maine, Institute for Health Policy, Maine Rural Health Research Center (Working Paper #23).

Brown, D. L., & Schafft, K. (2011). *Rural People and Communities.* Malden, MA: Polity Press.

Brown, D. L., & Swanson, L. (Eds.). (2003). *Challenges for Rural America in the Twenty-First Century.* University Park: Pennsylvania State University Press.

Carter, R. (2010). *Within Our Reach: Ending the Mental Health Crisis.* Emmaus, PA: Rodale Books.

Castle, E. (Ed.). (1995). The *Changing American Countryside: Rural People and Places.* Lawrence: University Press of Kansas.

Centers for Disease Control and Prevention (CDC). (December 18, 2015). Increases in drug and opioid overdose deaths—United States, 2000–2014. *Morbidity and Mortality Weekly Report,* 64(50), 1378–1382.

Centers for Disease Control and Prevention. (2011). *Public Health Action Plan to Integrate Mental Health Promotion and Mental Illness Prevention With Chronic Disease Prevention, 2011–2015.* Atlanta, GA: US Department of Health and Human Services.

Cloke, P., Marsden, T., & Mooney, P. H. (Eds.). (2006). *Handbook of Rural Studies.* Thousand Oaks, CA: Sage.

Coalition for Mental Health Reform (CMHR). (July 6, 2016). *Concerns With the Helping Families in Mental Health: Crisis Act of 2015—Passed in the House of Representatives.*

Cornell University. (2010). *Poverty, Local and Regional Government, Energy, Economic and Workforce Development, Agriculture and Food Systems.* Ithaca, NY. www.cornell.edu.

Danbom, D. H. (2006). *Born in the Country: A History of Rural America.* Baltimore: Johns Hopkins University Press.

Davidson, O. G. (1996). *Broken Heartland: The Rise of America's Rural Ghetto.* Iowa City: University of Iowa Press.

Duncan, C. (1999). *Worlds Apart: Why Poverty Persists in Rural America.* New Haven, CT: Yale University Press.

Elder, G., & Conger, R. (Eds.). (2000). *Children of the Land: Adversity and Success in Rural America.* Chicago: University of Chicago Press.

Flora, C.B., & Flora, J.L. (2008). *Rural Communities, Legacy and Change* (3rd ed.). Philadelphia, PA: Westview Press/Perseus Books.

Gamble, D. N., & Weil, M. (2010). *Community Practice Skills: Local to Global Perspectives.* New York: Columbia University Press.

Goldman, H. H., Buck, J. A., & Thompson, K. S., (2009). *Transforming Mental Health Services: Implementing the Federal Agenda for Change.* Arlington, VA: American Psychiatric Association.

Grantham, D. (June 1, 2015). National Association of County Behavioral Health and Developmental Disability Directors (NACBHDD). *Under the Microscope: Developing Effective Alternatives to Incarceration for Those With MH and SUD Conditions.* Washington, DC.

Grantham, D. (April 1, 2016). National Association of County Behavioral Health and Developmental Disability Directors (NACBHDD). Under the Microscope: *Salt Lake County's System of Care Thrives in Hostile Funding Environment.* Washington, DC.

Grantham, D. (July 1, 2016). National Association of County Behavioral Health and Developmental Disability Directors (NACBHDD). *Under the Microscope: A Single National Standard for Peer Specialist Certification.* Washington, DC.

Grantham, D. (February 1, 2017). National Association of County Behavioral Health and Developmental Disability Directors (NACBHDD). *The Challenge of Affordable Health Care: The ACA and Beyond.* Washington, DC.

Group for the Advancement of Psychiatry. (1995). *Mental Health in Remote Rural Developing Areas.* Washington, DC: American Psychiatric Press.

Hartley. D., Bird, D., Lambert, D., & Coffin, J. (November, 2002). *The Role of Community Mental Health Centers as Rural Safety Net Providers.* Portland: University of Southern Research Center. Maine, Edmund S. Muskie School of Working Paper #30.

Hartley, D., Ziller, E., Lambert, D., Loux, S., & Bird, D. (October, 2002). *State Licensure Laws and the Mental Health Professions: Implications For the Rural Mental Health Workforce.* Portland: University of Southern Maine, Edmund S. Muskie School of Public Service, Maine Rural Health Research Center (Working Paper #29).

Imhoff, D. (2012). *Food Fight: The Citizens Guide to the Next Food and Farm Bill.* Healdsburg, CA: Watershed Media.

Imig, A. (July 12, 2016). *Small But Mighty: Perspectives of Rural Mental Health Counselors.* The Professional Counselor. www.nbcc.org.

Jamison, J., & Blank, M. (2007). The role of clinical psychology in rural mental health services: Defining problems and developing solutions. *Clinical Psychology: Science and Practice*, 14, 283–298.

Kagan, R., & Schlosberg, S. (1989). *Families in Perpetual Crisis*. New York: W.W. Norton.

Kennedy, P. J. (2015). *A Common Struggle: A Personal Journey Through the Past and Future of Mental Illness and Addiction*. New York: Blue Rider Press.

Kim, N., Mickelson, J., Brenner, B., Haws, C., Yurgelun-Todd, D., & Renshaw, P. (September, 2010). Altitude, gun ownership, rural areas, and suicide. *American Journal of Psychiatry*. www.ncbi.nlm.nih.gov/pmc/articles/PMC4643668/

Layard, R., & Clark, D. M. (2015). *Thrive: How Better Mental Health Care Transforms Lives and Saves Money*. Princeton, NJ: Princeton University Press.

Lightburn, A., & Sessions, P. (2006). *Handbook of Community-Based Clinical Practice*. New York: Oxford University Press.

Manderscheid, R. (March 23, 2015). *Stigma Kills: On the Five "P's" of Inclusion and Social Justice*. www.nacbhdd.org.

Manderscheid, R. (June 7, 2016). Helping rural counties keep abreast of urban counterparts. *Behavioral Healthcare Magazine*. www.behavioral.net.

Manderscheid, R. (August 28, 2016). Last chance to pass mental health reform? *Behavioral Healthcare Magazine*. www.behavioral.net.

Manderscheid, R. (August 30, 2016). *Hillary Clinton Offers Excellent Mental Health Policy Proposals*. www.behavioral.net.

Manderscheid, R. (December 19, 2016). *Treatment and Housing for Persons With Serious Mental Illness*. www.naco.org.

Mental Health America. (August 29, 2016). *Statement by Paul Gionfriddo, President and CEO, Mental Health America*.

Mental Health and Rural America: 1994–2005. (2005). Washington, DC: Health Resources and Services Administration, Office of Rural Health Policy.

Meyer, D., Hamel-Lambert, J., Tice, C., Safran, S., Bolon, D., Rose-Grippa, K. (2005). Recruiting and retaining mental health professionals to rural communities: An interdisciplinary course in Appalachia. *Journal of Rural Health*, Winter, 21(1), 86–91.

Mohatt, D. F. (2016). *Rural Mental Health: Challenges and Opportunities Caring for the Country*. Boulder, CO: Western Interstate Commission for Higher Education.

Morris, J. (2009). Marriage and family therapists expand access to mental health services in rural areas. *Journal of Rural Community Psychology*, Summer, E12(1).

Morris, J. A. (1997). *Practicing Psychology in Rural Settings*. Washington, DC: American Psychological Association.

National Rural Health Association (October, 2008). *Government Affairs Office. Policy Position: Workforce Series—Rural Behavioral Health*. Washington, DC.

Neufeld, J., Case, R., Serricchio, M. (2012, Fall/Winter). *Walk-in Telemedicine Clinics Improve Access and Efficiency: A Program Evaluation From the Perspective of a Rural Community Mental Health Center*. Washington, DC: Rural Mental Health.

New Freedom Commission on Mental Health (2003). *Achieving the Promise: Transforming Mental Health Care in America*. Final. DHHS Pub. Co. SMA-03-3832. Rockville, MD.

Obama, B. (September 6, 2011). *Establishment of the White House Rural Council, Executive Order #13575.* Washington, DC: Office of the Federal Register. www.hsdl.org.

Office of the Surgeon General (US), Center for Mental Health Services (US), National Institute of Mental Health (US), Rockville (MD), Substance Abuse and Mental Health Services Administration (US). (August, 2001). *Mental Health Care for American Indians and Alaska Natives.*

Public Service, Maine Rural Health Research Center (PSMRHRC) (July, 2014). Working Paper #30. *Homeless in Rural America.* National Advisory Committee on Rural Health and Human Services. Retrieved from http://hrsa.gov/advisorycommittee/rural/publications.

Rainer, J. P. (2010). The road much less traveled: Treating rural and isolated clients. *Journal of Clinical Psychology: In Session,* 66(5), 475–478.

Rural Policy Research Institute. (2016). www.rupri.org.

Sawyer, D., Gale, J., & Lambert, D. (2006). *Rural and Frontier Mental and Behavioral health Care: Barriers, Effective Policy Strategies, and Best Practices.* Washington, DC: National Association for Rural Mental Health.

A Short History of the Farm Bill. (2016). *A Short History of the Farm Bill.* Arlington, VA: Farm Policy Facts. www.farmpolicyfacts.org.

Slama, K. (2004). Toward rural cultural competence. *Minnesota Psychologist,* 53(2), 6–13.

Smalley, K. B., Warren, J., & Rainer, J. (Eds.). (2012). *Rural Mental Health: Issues, Policies, and Best Practices.* New York: Springer.

Smalley, K. B., Yancey, C. T., Warren, J. C., Naufel, K., Ryan, R., & Pugh, J. L. (2010). Rural mental health and psychological treatment: A review for practitioners. *Journal of Clinical Psychology: In Session,* 66(5), 479–489.

Smith, A. (2003). Rural mental health counseling: One example of practicing what the research preaches. *Journal of Rural Community Psychology,* E6(2), Fall.

Stamm, B. H., (Ed.). (2003). *Rural Behavioral Health Care.* Washington, DC: American Psychological Association.

Thomas, A., Lowe, B., Fulkerson, G., & Smith, P. (2011). *Critical Rural Theory: Structure, Space, Culture.* New York: Lexington Books.

Vandiver, V. L. (2013). *Best Practices in Community Mental Health.* Chicago: Lyceum Books.

Weigel, D. (2009). *The Challenges of Rural Clinical Mental Health Counseling.* Weitz, Germany: VDM Verlag.

Wood, R. E. (2008). *Survival of Rural America: Small Victories and Bitter Harvests.* Lawrence: University Press of Kansas.

12 The Three "R's" of Schools in Rural Areas
Reassurance, Responsibility, and Resolution

Rural central schools are a natural setting for working with children and adolescents in rural America. Most rural schools house grades Pre-K through 12th grades. Rural areas have unique and increased busing needs and issues, with fewer resources. Research shows that the earlier we teach our children emotional literacy skills, the higher their functioning will be and in turn they can build resiliency. This chapter looks into adverse childhood experiences (ACEs), the President's New Freedom Commission's recommendations for school-aged children, and ways that the psychological and educational communities can collaborate for the benefit of working with rural children and their families.

According to the President's New Freedom Commission on Mental Health, "Children with serious emotional disturbances have the highest rates of school failure. Fifty percent of these students drop out of high school, compared to 30% of all students with disabilities."

Rural schools are most often "central" schools, being the only school in town and serving students in grades Pre-K through 12. Students between those ages ride on school buses together, often having rides of an hour or more. The fast-changing weather in many areas can make those runs even longer. Some students who live outside of Main Street can't play sports unless they have someone who will commit to the daily drop-offs and pick-ups after practice and games.

Many children in our country spend significant hours riding school buses, particularly in rural areas. The school bus environment is a unique combination of physical constraint, limited social opportunities, and varied ages. The psychology of the school bus experience is in and of itself fascinating. In a research article in the *Journal of Rural Community Psychology*, several factors were mentioned when students were asked about their experiences. Riders had to learn to deal with negative behaviors such as teasing and bullying, but many also used the constrained environment of the bus to develop friendships with students they may otherwise not have come into contact with. In many rural areas, students have pick-ups very early in the morning because of the distances traveled, which shortens their sleep cycle. Many parents expressed concern over young children's contact with older children and the potential for them to be exposed to drugs, violence, foul language, and sexual knowledge, causing them to grow up too fast. School consolidation, a concept that is gaining strength because of its cost-effectiveness, causes significant increases in the length of bus runs to and from schools. The school bus environment is a self-contained capsule that has the potential to be disastrous for many of our students. It needs to be considered carefully when dealing with the emotional health of our kids and the consolidating of schools in rural areas. The Kennedy Forum, founded by Congressman Patrick Kennedy of Rhode Island, son of Senator Ted Kennedy, has done a great deal of advocacy and research into issues in mental health including in our schools. The Forum believes that the poor academic performance in the United States as compared to other countries is largely due to a lack of early and ideal childhood interventions, especially in schools with large, low-income populations. Research in neuroscience proves that even the best teaching and curricula can have surprisingly little effect when a child's cognitive and emotional readiness to learn is not adequately addressed.

The Kennedy Forum also points out that research shows that a community approach to mental health is highly effective. It has also been consistently documented that bringing mental health services to a community is much more successful than having children and their families go outside their communities for services. This makes school systems the ideal location to meet the mental health needs of children and adolescents.

The Kennedy Forum suggests that by creating mental health systems within our schools that forge partnerships with community mental health professionals and researchers, we increase the likelihood of identifying students' emotional needs at earlier ages, provide pathways in developing innovative prevention and intervention programs, and create an integrative system of care so students have access to the kind of treatment needed when they need it and build the capacity to sustain mental health services over time. In order to accomplish these goals, they recommend several approaches. First, leadership on the national level needs to facilitate widespread adoption of evidence-based brain fitness executive function training while also integrating social emotional and brain literacy through the development widespread adoption of programs, tools, and resources. Second, they support a national brain health and fitness public awareness and advocacy campaign that extends into schools, communities, research, and the political arena. Third, we need state and federal policies that fund nationally required brain health and fitness implementation and assessment plans in early education through high school, including teacher trainings, with special funding for high-needs districts. In addition to use in schools, these should also be applied to citizens of all ages and socioeconomic status.

So how does a small rural school with limited funding and perhaps shrinking enrollment find the resources to provide these sorely needed services?

When the emotional needs of a child increase beyond what a school can provide, adequate resources must be made available within the rural communities. But you can't get blood from a stone in a rural area whose mental health resources are already stretched to the point of snapping.

Another benefit to housing a mental health program within rural schools is that school staff could then work with parents to increase their knowledge and understanding of social issues and mental illness so that they can become stronger advocates as a participating part of their child's treatment team. Such a program would be required to use evidence-based treatments, and implement emotional literacy and character education programs that become embedded in the core curriculum. These should teach, among other things, self-esteem, team building, and leadership training, as well as teach kids to be anti-bullying advocates. Schools all across America need to treat mental wellness as seriously as any other subject. If a child is not emotionally equipped, no amount of good teaching will reach him or her. Such programs would build student resiliency through providing greater understanding of the structure and function of the brain, some basic neuroscience, with attention given to brain fitness and positive ways students can maintain mental wellness and what to do if they are feeling angry, sad, or have low self-esteem. Emotional literacy education, or social/emotional as some in the field refer to it, also fosters self-confidence, resiliency, healing, and better self-control. Some of this education should be done directly in classrooms with the counselor teaching periodic lessons, but this information can also be taught in health and/or biology class.

Mental health must be given equal importance to physical health concerns. While students have regularly scheduled school physical examinations, mental screenings should be done as part of the exam. This would increase the likelihood that social, emotional, and behavioral issues can be discovered earlier, because we know that, left untreated, they have the ability to negatively impact all aspects of a child's life. Schools would have to identify the standardized assessment tools they will use and develop a system to protect confidentiality while streamlining communication between school personnel and community-based mental health providers

Most undergraduate and graduate education programs don't provide much in the way of training regarding social, emotional, and behavioral challenges with students. More professional development opportunities in these areas would provide teachers with tools and approaches to teach children emotional literacy skills. These trainings should include conflict resolution, de-escalation techniques, handling bullying incidents, ways to incorporate mindfulness into students' lives, and the impact of trauma on child development and learning. At the very least, all staff should be trained in psychological first aid and in non-violent crisis intervention. And like anywhere else, a positive atmosphere starts at the top with administrative support. Without support from administrators, even the best program will have limited results.

According to the Kennedy Forum, key points for sustainability of these programs include the following: school-based mental health programming must include ongoing assessment, data collection, progress monitoring, and program evaluation; identifying and implementing barriers to a comprehensive school-based mental health program; partnerships with universities will aid school districts in increasing funding through grant applications; limiting the number of students placed in the least restrictive environments allows for the redistribution of funding to district-based programming.

The Forum calls for some policy changes. For instance, on a local level, central school administrators should require mental health and emotional literacy programs by including them in school improvement plans and allocating appropriate funding. The federal government can mandate that educational institutions develop school-based mental health clinics, can increase federal funding to implement school-based mental health programs, and can also increase federal funding to states' systems of care to provide greater mental health services for children of all ages.

Adverse Childhood Experiences (ACEs) and Their Lingering Effects

Adverse childhood experiences (ACEs) is the all-encompassing term given to describe traumatic events experienced by a child such as abuse, neglect, loss, and the like. The effect on children from experiences like physical or emotional abuse, witnessing domestic violence, homelessness, and grief are similar to what soldiers undergo in combat. The part of the brain that controls the fight/flight/freeze response becomes temporarily larger, while the part of the brain that is responsible for memory, learning, and impulse control becomes temporarily smaller. So, it stands to reason that children who have undergone trauma without subsequent treatment have what I call an "emotional haze" around them, preventing them from learning and often from behaving appropriately. It is our responsibility as a society to see that our children receive the proper treatment they need and deserve. They are our future.

We need to focus on finding new ways to bring together the mental health and the educational communities to work toward the common goal of reducing health issues and barriers to learning, both academic and nonacademic. We all know that by addressing mental health issues in students, we improve their school performance, their social and emotional skills, and we ensure that they graduate ready to become fully contributing members of our society. Rural schools in particular must maintain a collaborative relationship with community resources in order to identify all students in need and ensure that they receive support. Schools must implement programs that emphasize prevention and early intervention while also promoting resiliency and self-advocacy. A central component of this approach would be universal screening at key transition points in elementary, middle, and high schools. These screenings would use evidence-based tools with clear procedural guidelines that also preserve the privacy of students. It is also vital that all school personnel are trained in youth mental health first aid.

The President's New Freedom Commission's Recommendations for Children

When the President's New Freedom Commission was formed in 2002, the committee's conclusion included goals and recommendations for mental health in America's schools, such as:

- Advance and implement a national campaign to reduce the stigma of seeking care and a national strategy for suicide prevention.
- Address mental health with the same urgency as physical health.
- Develop an individualized plan of care for every child with a serious emotional disturbance.
- Involve consumers and families in orienting the mental health system toward recovery.
- Align relevant federal programs to improve access and accountability for mental health services.
- Create a comprehensive state mental health plan.
- Protect and enhance the right of people with mental illness.
- Improve access to high-quality care that is culturally competent.
- Improve access to high-quality care in rural and geographically remote areas.
- Promote the mental health of young children.
- Improve and expand school mental health programs.
- Screen for co-occurring mental and substance use disorders and link with integrated treatment strategies.
- Screen for mental disorders in primary care across the lifespan and connect individuals to treatment and supports.
- Accelerate research to promote recovery and resilience and ultimately to cure and prevent mental illnesses.
- Advance evidence-based practices by using dissemination and demonstration projects and create a public-private partnership to guide their implementation.
- Improve and expand the workforce providing evidence-based mental health services and supports.
- Develop the knowledge base in four understudied areas: mental health disparities, long-term effects of medication, trauma, and acute care.
- Use health technology and telehealth to improve access and coordination of mental health care, especially for Americans in remote areas or in underserved populations.
- Develop and implement integrated electronic health record and personal health information system.

References

Bain, S. F. (November, 2010). Itinerant counseling services for rural communities: A win/win opportunity. *Journal of Rural Community Psychology*, E13(1).

Carr, P. J., & Kefalas, M. J. (2009). *Hollowing Out the Middle: The Rural Brain Drain and What It Means for America*. Boston: Beacon Press.

Carter, R. (2010). *Within Our Reach: Ending the Mental Health Crisis*. Emmaus, PA: Rodale Books.

Centers for Disease Control and Prevention (2011). *Public Health Action Plan to Integrate Mental Health Promotion and Mental Illness Prevention With Chronic Disease Prevention. 2011–2015*. Atlanta, GA: US Department of Health and Human Services.

Coalition for Mental Health Reform (CMHR). (July 6, 2016). *Concerns With the Helping Families in Mental Health Crisis Act of 2015—Passed in the House of Representatives*.

Cornell University. (2010). *Poverty, Local and Regional Government, Energy, Economic and Workforce Development, Agriculture and Food Systems*. Ithaca, NY. www.cornell.edu.

Danbom, D. H. (2006). *Born in the Country: A History of Rural America*. Baltimore: Johns Hopkins University Press.

Davidson, O. G. (1996). *Broken Heartland: The Rise of America's Rural Ghetto*. Iowa City: University of Iowa Press.

Elder, G., & Conger, R. (Eds.). (2000). *Children of the Land: Adversity and Success in Rural America*. Chicago: University of Chicago Press.

Federal Office of Rural Health Policy (FORHP). (March 17, 2017). *Special Announcement—CDC on Rural Children and Mental Health*.

Federal Office of Rural Health Policy. (April 5, 2017). *FORHP Announcements. What's New*. Washington, DC.

Fitchen, J. (1991). *Endangered Spaces, Enduring Places*. Boulder, CO: Westview Press.

Ginsberg, L. H. (2005). Social *Work in Rural Communities* (4th ed.). Alexandria, VA: Council on Social Work Education.

Gladding, S. T. (1997). *Community and Agency Counseling*. Upper Saddle River, NJ: Prentice-Hall.

Goldman, H. H., Buck, J. A., & Thompson, K. S. (2009). *Transforming Mental Health Services: Implementing the Federal Agenda for Change*. Arlington, VA: American Psychiatric Association.

Hartley, D., Bird, D., Lambert, D., & Coffin, J. (November, 2002). *The Role of Community Mental Health Centers as Rural Safety Net Providers*. Portland: University of Southern Maine, Edmund S. Muskie School of Public Service, Maine Rural Health Research Center (Working Paper #30).

Hartley, D., Ziller, E., Lambert, D., Loux, S., & Bird, D. (October, 2002). *State Licensure Laws and the Mental Health Professions: Implications For the Rural Mental Health Workforce*. Portland: University of Southern Maine, Edmund S. Muskie School of Public Service, Maine Rural Health Research Center (Working Paper #29).

Henderson, B. (2009, Summer). The school bus: A neglected children's environment. *Journal of Rural Community Psychology*, E12(1).

Jamison, J., & Blank, M. (2007). The role of clinical psychology in rural mental health services: Defining problems and developing solutions. *Clinical Psychology: Science and Practice*, 14, 283–298.

Joseph, G., Strain, P., & Ostrosky, M.M. (September, 2005). *Fostering Emotional Literacy in Young Children: Labeling Emotions.* Center on the Social and Emotional Foundations For Early Learning. HHS: Child Care and Head Start Bureaus.

Kennedy Forum. (2016). *Navigating the New Frontier of Mental Health and Addiction: A Guide for the 115th Congress.* www.parityregistry.org, www.thekennedyforum.org; www.paritytrack.org.

Kennedy, P.J. (2015). *A Common Struggle: A Personal Journey Through the Past and Future of Mental Illness and Addiction.* New York: Blue Rider Press.

Morris, J.A. (1997). *Practicing Psychology in Rural Settings.* Washington, DC: American Psychological Association.

New Freedom Commission on Mental Health. (2003). *Achieving the Promise: Transforming Mental Health Care in America.* Final. DHHS Pub. Co. SMA-03-3832. Rockville, MD.

Olfman, S. (2015). *The Science and Pseudoscience of Children's Mental Health.* Santa Barbara, CA: Praeger.

Paceley, M. (July 21, 2016). *Study Determines Needs of LGBTQ Youth in Rural Areas.* www.news.ku.edu/2016/05/06/study-determines-needs-lgbtq-youth-rural-areas-how- social-workers-communities-can-help.

Parental Incarceration's Impact on Children's Health. (May, 2012). The New York Initiative for Children of Incarcerated Parents, The Osborne Association. NYInitiative@osborneny.org.

Safran, M.A., Mays, R.A., Jr., Huang, L. N., McCuan, R., Pham, P. K., Fisher, S. K., McDuffie, K.Y., & Trachtenberg, A. (November, 2009). Mental health disparities. *American Journal of Public Health*, 99(11), 1962–1966.

Sawyer, D., Gale, J., & Lambert, D. (2006). *Rural and Frontier Mental and Behavioral Health Care: Barriers, Effective Policy Strategies, and Best Practices.* Washington, DC: National Association for Rural Mental Health.

Slovac, K., & Singer, M. (2002, February). Children and violence: Findings and implications from a rural community. *Child & Adolescent Social Work Journal*, 19(1), 35–56.

Smalley, K.B., Warren, J., & Rainer, J. (Eds.). (2012). *Rural Mental Health: Issues, Policies, and Best Practices.* New York: Springer.

Smalley, K.B., Yancey, C.T., Warren, J.C., Naufel, K., Ryan, R., & Pugh, J.L. (2010). Rural mental health and psychological treatment: A review for practitioners. *Journal of Clinical Psychology: In Session*, 66(5), 479–489.

Smith, A. (2003). Rural mental health counseling: One example of practicing what the research preaches. *Journal of Rural Community Psychology*, E6(2), Fall.

Stamm, B.H. (Ed.). (2003). *Rural Behavioral Health Care.* Washington, DC: American Psychological Association.

Taubenheim, A., & Tiano, J. (2012). Rationale and modifications for implementing parent-child interaction therapy with rural Appalachian parents. *Rural Mental Health*, Fall/Winter.

Todey, J. (2009). Providing learning supports through school/community collaborations. *National Association for Rural Mental Health Newsletter*, 1(2), 1–6.

13 Substance Abuse in Rural Areas

We are living in the midst of the worst drug epidemic in American history, with no end in sight. How did it come to be, and what can we do about it? Couple that with alcohol abuse, which causes nearly double the number of fatal car crashes in rural areas, and you have a problem that is truly unprecedented. Rural residents have higher rates of substance abuse but are less likely to utilize treatment options. Many non-violent drug- and alcohol-related arrests lead to incarceration, which often provides little or no rehabilitation. Our prisons are filled to bursting and recidivism rates are high. This chapter surveys several of the most popular drugs in the epidemic and some government interventions, treatment methods, and case studies.

Prevalence, Causes, and Risk Factors

- OxyContin prescriptions for chronic pain rose from 670,000 in 1997 to 6.2 million in 2002.
- Every day, 246 people die from suicide or drug overdoses.
- Approximately one in five adults aged 18 or older—43.6 million Americans—experiences mental illness in a year. About half of this number—21.5 million Americans—has a substance addiction. This public health crisis costs the nation at least $467 billion annually in health care, lost earnings, and public disability payments. Yet over half of the individuals with a mental illness do not receive medically necessary treatment services. Even more astounding, 90% of Americans with a substance addiction do not receive appropriate care. Inadequate access to medically necessary treatment is partly responsible for the disease and economic burden attributable to these illnesses (Kennedy Guide for Congress).
- The opioid epidemic took more than 33,000 lives in calendar year 2015 (www.nacbhd.org).

Many studies show that in most rural areas of the United States, alcohol is the primary substance abused, followed by marijuana, stimulants, opioids, and cocaine. Most heroin users are introduced to the drug as an alternative to the illicit use of prescription painkillers and the like, because heroin is more readily available and affordable. Results vary as to the overall prevalence of alcohol and drug abuse in rural versus urban areas. It has repeatedly been shown in some studies to be comparable between rural and urban populations. In many other studies it has been shown to be disproportionately higher in rural areas, with suicide showing higher rates in rural areas as well. It has been estimated that about 40% of mentally ill rural residents have a comorbid substance use disorder, which complicates service provision.

Mental disorders and substance abuse disorders often co-occur for adults and children. Evidence-based practices have been established for treating these co-occurring disorders. However, there is little research on the incidence, prevalence, and etiology of co-occurring disorders in rural populations. Thus, the field lacks an understanding of the need and how to tailor these evidence-based practices to treat persons with co-occurring disorders in rural areas. State efforts to improve mental health and substance abuse service systems cannot overlook the fragmented data systems that reinforce the historical separateness of the various systems of care. These separate systems have specific approaches to treatment, and there are distinct funding streams for state mental health, substance abuse, and Medicaid agencies. Transforming mental health and substance abuse services in the United States depends on resolving issues that underlie separate treatment systems—access barriers, uneven quality, disjointed coordination, and information across agencies and providers.

In 2014, President Obama nominated Michael Botticelli to the position of director of the White House Office of National Drug Control Policy, making him the first person with addiction to hold the position. We should be continuing this trend, as who understands the nuances of drug treatment and recovery better than someone who has lived it?

At least part of the increased use of methamphetamines in rural areas is due to the low cost of manufacturing them, and the fact that they can be made anywhere, including the kitchen sink. Because rural areas have lower population density, increased isolation with deserted barns, farms and homes on remote roads, people have greater privacy while manufacturing the drug. According to *Rural Mental Health*, in addition to the severe physiological effects such as poor physical health and acute and long-term psychological and behavioral problems and personal effects such as family strife and child neglect, unsatisfactory work performance, and criminal behavior—effects suffered by people who are addicted to methamphetamines—meth abuse wreaks havoc on rural families and children, economies, law enforcement, social services, and the environment. The family effects of meth abuse include exposure to toxic chemicals or contaminated foods from home-based meth production. Societal effects include the economic burden put onto rural schools, hospitals, emergency rooms, human service agencies, and the legal and criminal justice systems in coping with the consequences of meth abuse. From an environmental point of view, the by-products of meth production include up to 5 pounds of toxic waste that filters into local water systems, soil, property, and buildings, causing contamination. These by-products can also cause serious risk of fire, explosion, and exposure to hazardous chemicals. Small rural communities frequently do not have the resources to address these problems. Ecological or environmental models of prevention that focus on the entire community have a better chance of success.

Alcohol

The rate of fatal motor vehicle crashes in which alcohol was a factor is nearly double in rural areas than urban areas. In 2013, there were 10,076 US fatalities from alcohol-impaired related car accidents; rural areas accounted for 54% of these. In addition, 31% of all rural car accidents were alcohol related (Traffic Safety Facts).

Many states are gradually implementing stricter driving while intoxicated (DWI) laws, stiffer penalties for those who are caught, and tougher sentencing for repeat offenders. There are some innovative solutions on the horizon such as the availability of "safe cabs" to call as needed, however these options can be expensive.

The Maine Rural Health Research Center published a study in 2012, the results of which indicated that binge drinking is more common among rural youth aged 12–13 than among urban youth of the same age. The study suggests that teens who begin drinking alcohol at an earlier age may engage in problem drinking as they get older. In surveys, rural teens reported higher rates of binge drinking and DWI than their urban peers. They cited several additional characteristics influencing the increased underage drinking and binge drinking occurrence. These include lower levels of parental disapproval, higher tolerance for alcohol use, increased availability of alcohol in households with higher income levels, easier access to alcohol at family events, and a greater number of adults willing to purchase alcohol for underage teens. In general, high levels of risky behavior are usually correlated to low levels of protective factors and prevention.

So what can be done to alleviate the problem? Community education and the public health model are a great starting point. Engaging the whole community is a critical piece. There are numerous civic and religious organizations that want to help with the drug and alcohol issues that plague their communities, stretching already thin rural resources. The Maine Rural Health Research Center study suggested that first and foremost, parental influence is a protective factor against alcohol use. Family-centered prevention programs work to improve knowledge and skills of residents of all ages related to substance use as well as teaching communication skills. Schools are an important facet of the community and can play an important role in helping discourage teens from substance use and abuse. Schools are a stable, supportive environment for students where they should feel cared for by faculty and staff. Children who are successful in school are less likely to drink alcohol. Religious facilities also play an important role in influencing teens and families. According to the above study, rural teens are more likely to participate in church-related events and could use activities focused on substance abuse prevention. Other community institutions that could help with the education process are libraries, arts organizations, social service agencies, mental health clinics, and many more. Rural areas need to think outside the box in terms of setting up programs that everyone buys into.

Research has shown that rural residents are able to abstain from drinking more than urban and suburban residents; however, among those who do drink, rural residents were more likely to abuse alcohol and drink excessive amounts compared to their counterparts. Alcoholics Anonymous and its related 12-step programs are widespread in all parts of the country, and are largely successful in encouraging and supporting recovery. I would like to see some alternative programs spreading through the countryside, as there is no one-size-fits-all approach to such a complex problem.

The Opioid Epidemic

The United States is experiencing a wide ranging drug and opioid crisis that shows all signs of continuing to grow in scope and severity. It is truly an unprecedented epidemic. According to the Department of Health and Human Services (HHS), in 2015 more than 33,000 Americans died of an overdose involving a prescription or illicit opioid, and more than two million individuals had an opioid use disorder. HHS launched its Opioid Initiative in partnership with state and local governments, health care professionals, and other key stakeholders, and has taken significant steps to improve opioid prescribing practices, increase the availability and use of naloxone to reverse opioid overdoses, and expand access to medication-assisted treatment with methadone, buprenorphine, or naloxone to be coupled with appropriate psychological services. The HHS has also continued to prioritize reducing stigma and prevention, treatment, and parity for people needing care for mental health and substance use disorders. The success of these strategies is largely determined on the basis of health insurance coverage. What that means is that our nation's best shot at reversing the opioid epidemic and providing needed care for opioid use disorders, others substance use disorders, and mental illness depends on the continued success of the Affordable Care Act (ACA).

It has become almost impossible to find an individual or a family that hasn't been touched by the drug epidemic. According to a Kaiser Family Foundation report, more than 44% of Americans know someone who has been addicted to prescription painkillers. In addition to the lives lost, the epidemic incurs $72 billion in health costs each year. Among the reasons for the explosion in drug use, especially in rural areas, is that heroin and meth replaced the economic base in Appalachia when the steel mills went bust, the coal industry began to shrink, and prisons and nuclear plants moved into many areas; these events set the stage for these drugs to become the basis for a new economy. The opioid epidemic is non-partisan and non-discriminatory, and has swept across the country with disregard for socioeconomic status or geographic location. It is sometimes disguised as a serious public health epidemic, and other times masked as a political issue.

In most states, the opioid epidemic has grown exponentially, which caused prisons to fill to the point of bursting. There, inmates with addiction issues were channeled through the penal system rather than given a chance at rehabilitation and therapy on the outside. The success rate for staying clean after release is extremely low, with the root causes of the addiction still intact. Most resources cite the success rate for kicking the habit as 1 in 10 upon discharge, and returning back to their familiar surroundings. Recent brain research has shown that it takes the brain far longer to recover from the ravages of drug use than the average person with addiction issues spends in the average drug rehabilitation program, which is usually several weeks to a month or two. The drug issue has advanced so much that in the past few years a decarceration movement has grown from the grassroots up. It is now on the federal agenda, with more lawmakers signing on to it all the time.

Compared to urban residents, rural residents have higher rates of substance abuse, but studies show that they are less likely to utilize drug treatment options. The vast majority of rural residents live in counties that do not have any detox facilities. Very often, law enforcement or emergency departments provide the initial detoxification services. Generally, the greater the distance one has to travel in order to receive substance abuse treatment of any kind, the lower the completion rates. The lack of facilities also provides a hardship for families who must drive long distances in order to visit and support their loved one while in residential treatment, and patients who have had their driver's licenses revoked are also at a loss to access these services. More research is needed in order to determine whether or not lack of access to substance abuse sites is the main obstacle, and how much a part stigma plays in their lack of participation in treatment. A national survey on drug use and health found that rural residents are more likely to use drugs like cocaine, methamphetamines, and stimulants compared to those from urban areas.

In 2013, approximately one in nine youth ages 12–17 were current alcohol users, regardless of which setting they lived in. According to a 2012 report from the Substance Abuse and Mental Health Services Administration (SAMHSA), rural admissions to substance abuse facilities were more likely than urban admissions to report primary abuse of alcohol. Urban admissions were more likely than rural admissions to report primary abuse of heroin or cocaine. Many schools, colleges, and universities have significantly increased the number of drug-related programs on their campuses, and some have even started recovery dorms. Much more research needs to be done in these areas in order to educate and hopefully prevent drug usage.

Mental disorders and substance abuse disorders are often comorbid for both children and adults. However, there is little research on the incidence, prevalence, and etiology of co-occurring disorders in rural populations. Therefore, we have little understanding of how we can improve our treatment for this population in rural areas. Much more research is urgently needed in this area.

Among the drugs included in the opioid epidemic is fentanyl, a synthetic opiate painkiller, which is being mixed with heroin to increase its potency. Very often, those who take it are unaware that it is mixed in with their heroin. Fentanyl can be deadly at very low doses and comes in several forms including powder, blotter paper, pills, and spray. The drug also poses significant threat to law enforcement and emergency workers and first responders who should be aware of any kind of exposure. Symptoms include respiratory depression or arrest, drowsiness, disorientation, sedation, pinpoint pupils, and clammy skin. The onset of the symptoms is usually within minutes of exposure.

Carfentanil is a synthetic opioid that is 10,000 times more potent than morphine and 100 times more potent than fentanyl, which is itself 50 times more potent than heroin. Immediate medical attention should be sought if there is any skin or breath contact with either drug, as it can be absorbed through the skin. Naloxone can be administered in larger than usual doses to combat either of these drugs.

Through the Cures Act of 2016, billions of dollars will be provided to each state to help combat the opioid and drug epidemic. Read more about the Cures Act in Chapter 2.

In May 2017, President Trump appointed New Jersey Governor Chris Christie to lead a bipartisan group of lawmakers, creating his White House Commission. The commission's task is to seek solutions to fight the opioid epidemic. Included on the task force is former Representative Patrick Kennedy, a champion for mental health services and parity. In the fall of 2016, just weeks before the election, Trump addressed a group of opioid stakeholders in New Hampshire by saying, "We will give people struggling with addiction access to the help they need. I would dramatically expand access to treatment slots." Six months later, mental health activists complained that it took too long to set up the task force, and in May 2017, reports broke that the White House planned to virtually eliminate the Office of National Drug Control Policy by cutting its budget by 94% (Manderscheid 5/11/17).

The Morphine Element

According to Sam Quinones in *Dreamland*, what gave the morphine molecule its immense power was that it evolved somehow to fit, key in lock, into the receptors that all mammals, especially humans, have in their brains and spines. The so-called mu-opioid receptors—which create pleasure sensations when they come into contact with endorphins produced naturally by the body—were especially welcoming to the morphine molecule. The receptor combines with endorphins to give us those glowing feelings we might feel at the sight of an infant or the feel of a furry puppy. The morphine molecule overwhelms the receptor, creating a far more intense euphoria than anything we come by naturally.

According to Coop in his interview with Quinones, during the torturous withdrawal from the drug, when someone stops ingesting it, the morphine molecule acts like a child having a tantrum. The same molecule that provided unprecedented joy causes the complete opposite effect when it is the only such molecule left. Most drugs are easily reduced to water-soluble glucose in the human body, which then expels them. The morphine molecule rebels by refusing to turn into glucose, and it remains in the body rather than being expelled.

Coop adds that researchers still don't understand why this happens. It's as if these molecules have a strong mind of their own. Thousands of other drugs in the world are broken down by the body and expelled. Morphine is different, and can be considered diabolical in this way.

Treatment Methods

The idea behind the Harrison Act of 1914 was to build a "narcotic farm" to house thousands of people with addiction issues. Sam Quinones describes its uniqueness as both a prison and a treatment center that remained in operation for over 40 years. The farm stressed outdoor work as addiction therapy. Inmates milked cows and raised crops such as tomatoes and wheat to supply the institution with food. In addition, there was a canning plant, a radio repair service, and a dental lab that made false teeth. Administrators believed that recreation was therapy. Patients played basketball and tennis; the farm had a golf course, a bowling alley, and basket weaving classes. For years the farm was the world's foremost center of addiction research, but in spite of its monumental effort, it never graduated much more than 10% of their patients to true recovery.

In my opinion, 12-step programs are terrific, but I would like to see the rise of an alternative philosophy. Having nothing available but 12-step programs is a one-size-fits-all approach. Alcoholics Anonymous (AA) and all its related programs are often found in rural areas; however, during this time of opioid and other rampant substance abuse, Narcotics Anonymous (NA) is rarely found. Often those wanting to attend an NA meeting must drive very long distances. We need to encourage communities to take on the NA challenge and create meetings in every rural area. Aside from being a low-cost resource, it creates an alternative sense of community and healing.

Another serious shortage of resources needed to help heal substance abusers in rural areas are residential treatment facilities, detox beds, and long-term-care. The creation of these badly needed services would not only help people recover, but would create jobs and boost local economies.

According to *Rural Mental Health*, in 2006 only 9% of all 13,600 treatment facilities in the United States were located in a rural county not adjacent to an urban county, with nearly 80% of facilities located in urban areas. Therefore, fewer inpatient and residential beds are located in rural areas (29.7 beds per 100,000) compared to urban areas (45.8 beds per 100,000). Unfortunately, the vast majority of rural residents (82%) live in a county without a detox provider, and we are in the midst of a major drug crisis in America. Almost all opioid treatment programs (programs that use methadone and other medications to treat heroin and other opiate addictions) are located in urban areas.

Successful prevention programs and initiatives in rural areas include:

- Targeting school-aged children, both in schools and the community
- Combining strategies focused on the individual with environmental strategies
- Engaging youth in program design and communication strategies
- Engaging communities, including retail outlets and law enforcement
- When possible, coordinating local interventions with statewide or multi-tribal campaigns.

Rural Matters: Hungry to Be Full

Dark hair and blue eyes is a rare and beautiful combination. On a 4-year-old girl, it is heartbreaking when those bright blue eyes become teary and the tip of her nose turns red. When she smiles, her dimples make her eyes shine, and when she's angry, those blue eyes seem to turn smoky gray. She has lived in foster care since she was just over a year old, and that is her normal. She refers to her current foster mom as "mommy" and to her foster siblings as brothers and sisters. It is an atypical family doing typical things together.

She was brought into foster care because her birth mom was addicted to heroin. At the age of 24, she had her baby and now, at age 28, she has been addicted for more than three years. The baby's father tried to be involved initially, but he worked long hours, leaving the mother to tend to the baby alone. He admitted to the social services caseworker that although he loved the baby, he was glad to get out of feeding, bathing, and diaper changing. As boring as his custodial job was, he would rather be at work most of his waking hours. Besides, he and his girlfriend had a stormy relationship at best. He hit her once, throwing her hard against the living room wall, giving her a huge black bruise around her left eye and the side of her face. She had taken a photograph of it with her cell phone and showed it to the caseworker after she reported him to the police. She turned down the offer of an order of protection and continued to live with him as if nothing happened. She did love him, but was afraid she would have nowhere to live and no money to buy food and other necessities if they broke up. And if he was arrested, it would jeopardize his job as a custodian at the college. Domestic violence was one of the grounds for dismissal from his job.

The baby was normal developmentally, with no signs of a delay in any area. Mom became depressed and refused to see anyone for help. She wouldn't consider taking an antidepressant; she didn't want drugs in her system at that time. So the depression snowballed, as depression is apt to do, and it was a long, sad winter for her and the baby alone in that tiny apartment on the second floor. The couple had one car, which he needed in order to get to and from work. At night when he got home, it was either too late or she was too tired to go for a ride anywhere, or the roads were snowy and icy.

One day the downstairs neighbor came upstairs to borrow some coffee, and couldn't help but notice the sad demeanor that permeated the apartment as mom sat with the lights off in the dark while the baby was in the playpen. Unbeknownst to the sad young mother, her neighbor used the coffee as an excuse to come into the apartment to see why the baby was crying for so long. Next to her were cigarettes burned to the butt in the ashtray. She lit them and lost the focus to smoke them. She lit one up as the neighbor sat herself down next to her on the couch, and it was then that the needle tracks on her inside right forearm became apparent. She self-consciously pulled her sleeves down, but they weren't long enough to cover it all.

When the police came later that evening, she was so out of it she couldn't even deny she was using. She could barely make sense of what was happening. They hoisted her out of the apartment and carried the baby right behind to be taken to a foster home.

The jail cell was cold and damp when she awoke the next afternoon. She couldn't figure out why she was there and her head throbbed. Sitting with knees bent and her hands over her face she had a vague recollection of her neighbor sitting near her and the baby being in the playpen, but that was all. It didn't even dawn on her to wonder where the baby was.

That baby grew up in foster care from that point on. Her father signed over his parental rights to her. He signed on the dotted line as mechanically as if he were paying a bill. That baby's eyes grew a brighter and brighter blue the longer she was in foster care, but the emptiness she felt inside herself kept growing, causing an insatiable hunger for love and affection. She was hungry to be full.

While working with me she denied most of her feelings. Other people feel like that but not me, she would say. I told her that it's OK for people to feel sad or mad, that most of us do at different times. She nodded and continued playing mommy to the baby dolls. She changed their diapers and fed them before putting them in the playpen. "I want you to read me that book about the Runaway Bunny," she demanded. "You know the one where the baby runs away and the mommy comes running after her to find her," she added. I know the one. I know the one indeed.

Rural Matters: Hump of the Moon

What follows is a phone conversation between me and a social services caseworker, discussing a case we have in common that involves a 5-year-old foster child.

CW: This child has been in therapy for 2 1/2 years already with little change. You've been seeing her for almost a year of it. I just don't see much in the way of progress. You're going to have to be more aggressive in your treatment. Her foster mother reports that she is having more bad days than good. She has tantrums that sometimes last hours, hits herself, bangs her head on the wall, hits and kicks other kids, and is jealous whenever the foster mother pays attention to anyone else, even her grown daughter. She tried to hurt the cat recently, and can sometimes be verbally defiant in school and day care. Something has to change and change quickly, or this child is going to have to start over at a new placement if I can even find one.

ME: Well, I do see progress, although it's subtle. This child is 5 years old and has lived in as many houses. We know she witnessed domestic violence as an infant and maybe as a toddler. We know her parents neglected her enough for her to be taken from them and put into foster care. What we don't know is what other kinds of stresses she has experienced. Sexual or physical abuse? Lack of adequate food? Being locked in closets? So many of our foster kids have been through those things and it changes the brain's chemistry to be under prolonged stress like that.

CW: Her mother was a drug addict. I believe her father was too, although he was able to keep a job and take care of business enough to be able to have continued visits with her until a few years ago. Does she ever mention him?

ME: No, she never mentions her dad. She does talk about her birth mom, though. Quite often. What I'm trying to do is teach her some emotional literacy skills. It's like putting tools in a child's toolbox, and the younger we do this with all kids, the better will be able to and manage their feelings. It's things like accepting emotions and knowing appropriate ways of releasing them. For example, I often tell young kids, "It's OK to be angry but it's not OK to hit or kick others," and then I work with them on appropriate ways to express anger.

CW: Give me an example of some appropriate ways of expressing anger.

ME: Well, hitting a pillow, listening to soothing music or sounds, taking deep belly breaths, crying, drawing—there are many ways kids can release dark emotions. With this child, part of the job I have is to help her with self-esteem. Hers is understandably rock bottom. I praise every good thing she does, however small. I encourage her, when she does a good job, to understand that not only am I proud of her, but that she can be proud of herself. She is showing that she understands how good it feels to feel good about yourself.

CW: Well, I guess I can ask for approval for you to see her for another month or two.

ME: That would be great. But again, we're looking at a long-term treatment plan here. This child has experienced so much in her short life and we owe it to her to give her the opportunity to heal. She has so many strengths other kids in her situation don't have and those are to her advantage.

CW: What do you consider her strengths?

ME: She's very smart intellectually, has an extensive vocabulary, and is very capable of loving others, even though she doesn't always show empathy. This child acts out in an attempt to control a life she has had absolutely no control over.

CW: You're the only one who is feeling optimistic about her. We all know what happens to these kids as they get older and end up in residential care or worse on the street . . .

ME: Wait—she is only 5. If we work hard enough with her now, we have a long time before she's a teenager to really reach her and teach her the skills she needs to avoid those fates . . .

CW: I'll call you back and let you know whether or not I get approval for her to continue seeing you [she hangs up the phone].

I hang up reluctantly, knowing in my heart I am beginning to reach this child who likes coming to her sessions. I also know that this foster placement is potentially an adoptive home for her, and I want so much for her to have that opportunity. She loves her foster mother. I wander onto the back porch where the air is cooler after a thunderstorm. The sky has cleared and on the horizon, the rising moon hangs crooked.

References

Bagalman, E. (2016). *The Helping Families in Mental Health Crisis Reform Act of 2016*. Washington, DC: Congressional Research Service.

Brown, D. L., & Schafft, K. (2011). *Rural People and Communities*. Malden, MA: Polity Press.

Carter, R. (2010). *Within Our Reach: Ending the Mental Health Crisis*. Emmaus, PA: Rodale Books.

Census.gov/geo/tiger/glossry2.html.

Centers for Disease Control and Prevention (CDC) (December 18, 2015). Increases in Drug and Opioid Overdose Deaths— United States, 2000-2014. *Morbidity and Mortality Weekly Report*, 64(50), 1378–1382.

Cloke, P., Marsden, T., & Mooney, P. H. (Eds.). (2006). *Handbook of Rural Studies*. Thousand Oaks, CA: Sage.

Coalition for Mental Health Reform. (July 6, 2016).*Concerns With the Helping Families in Mental Health: Crisis Act of 2015—Passed in the House of Representatives.*

Davidson, O. G. (1996). *Broken Heartland: The Rise of America's Rural Ghetto*. Iowa City: University of Iowa Press.

Doherty, G., & Jones, J. (2013). *Crisis in the American Heartland: Challenges of Returning Veterans*. (Volume 2). Rocky, MT: DMH Institute Press.

Goldman, H. H., Buck, J. A., & Thompson, K. S. (2009). *Transforming Mental Health Services: Implementing the Federal Agenda for Change*. Arlington, VA: American Psychiatric Association.

Goleman, D. (2009). *Ecological Intelligence*. New York; Broadway Books.

Grantham, D. (June 1, 2015). National Association of County Behavioral Health and Developmental Disability Directors. *Under the Microscope: Developing Effective Alternatives to Incarceration for those with MH and SUD Conditions*. Washington, DC.

Grantham, D. (April 1, 2016). National Association of County Behavioral Health and Developmental Disability Directors. *Under the Microscope: Salt Lake County's System of Care Thrives in Hostile Funding Environment.* Washington, DC.

Grantham, D. (February 1, 2017). National Association of County Behavioral Health and Developmental Disability Directors. *The Challenge of Affordable Health Care: The ACA and Beyond.* Washington, DC.

Hartley. D., Bird, D., Lambert, D., & Coffin, J. (November, 2002). *The Role of Community Mental Health Centers as Rural Safety Net Providers.* Portland: University of Southern Maine, Edmund S. Muskie School of Public Service, Maine Rural Health Research Center (Working Paper #30).

Intimate Partner Violence in Rural America. (March, 2015). *National Advisory Committee on Rural Health and Human Services.* Retrieved from www.hrsa.gov/advisorycommittee/rural/publications.

Kagan, R., & Schlosberg, S. (1989). *Families in Perpetual Crisis.* New York: W.W. Norton.

Kegler, S.R., Stone, D.M., & Holland, K.M. (2017). Trends in suicide by level of urbanization—United States, 1999–2015. *MMWR Morbidity Mortality Weekly Report,* 66, 270–273. https://doi.org/10.15585/mmwr.mm6610a2

Kennedy Forum. (2016). *Navigating the New Frontier of Mental Health and Addiction: A Guide for the 115th Congress.* www.parityregistry.org; www.thekennedyforum.org; www.paritytrack.org.

Kennedy, P.J. (2015). *A Common Struggle: A Personal Journey Through the Past and Future of Mental Illness and Addiction.* New York: Blue Rider Press.

Kim, N., Mickelson, J., Brenner, B., Haws, C., Yurgelun-Todd, D., & Renshaw, P. (September, 2010). Altitude, gun ownership, rural areas, and suicide. *American Journal of Psychiatry.* www.ncbi.nlm.nih.gov/pmc/articles/PMC4643668/

Lightburn, A., & Sessions, P. (2006). *Handbook of Community-Based Clinical Practice.* New York: Oxford University Press.

Manderscheid, R. (March 23, 2015). *Stigma Kills: On the Five "P's" of Inclusion and Social Justice.* www.nacbhdd.org.Merica, D. (May 10, 2017). *Trump Fills Out Commission Tasked With Fighting Opioid Abuse.* www.cnn.com.

Manderscheid, R. (June 7, 2016). Helping rural counties keep abreast of urban counterparts. *Behavioral Healthcare Magazine.* www.behavioral.net.

Mohatt, D. F. (2016). *Rural Mental Health: Challenges and Opportunities Caring for the Country.* Boulder, CO: Western Interstate Commission for higher Education.

New Freedom Commission on Mental Health. (2003). *Achieving the Promise: Transforming Mental Health Care in America.* Final. DHHS Pub. Co. SMA-03-3832. Rockville, MD.

Office of the Surgeon General (US), Center for Mental Health Services (US), National Institute Of Mental Health (US), Rockville (MD), Substance Abuse and Mental Health Services Administration (US). (August, 2001). *Mental Health Care for American Indians and Alaska Natives.*

Office of the Assistant Secretary for Planning and Evaluation. Department of Health and Human Services. (January 11, 2017). *Continuing Progress on the Opioid Epidemic: The Role Of the Affordable Care Act.* Rockville, MD.

Quinones, S. (2015). *Dream Land: The True Tale of America's Opiate Epidemic.* New York: Bloomsbury Press.

Ramirez-Ferrero, E. (2005). *Troubled Fields: Men, Emotions and the Crisis in American Farming*. New York: Columbia University Press.

Ranier, J. P. (2010). The road much less traveled: Treating rural and isolated clients. *Journal of Clinical Psychology: In Session*, 66(5), 475–478.

Reding, N. (2009). *Methland: The Death and Life of an American Small Town*. New York: Bloomsbury.

Rural Mental Health and Substance Abuse Toolkit. (2016). www.ruralhealthinfo.org/community-health/substance-abuse.

Sawyer, D., Gale, J., & Lambert, D. (2006). *Rural and Frontier Mental and Behavioral Health Care: Barriers, Effective Policy Strategies, and Best Practices*. Washington, DC: National Association for Rural Mental Health.

Smalley, K. B., Warren, J., & Rainer, J. (Eds.). (2012). *Rural Mental Health: Issues, Policies, and Best Practices*. New York: Springer.

Smalley, K. B., Yancey, C. T., Warren, J. C., Naufel, K., Ryan, R., & Pugh, J. L. (2010). Rural mental health and psychological treatment: A review for practitioners. *Journal of Clinical Psychology: In Session*, 66(5), 479–489.

Stamm, B. H. (Ed.). (2003). *Rural Behavioral Health Care*. Washington, DC: American Psychological Association.

Stone, D. M., Holland, K. M., Bartholow, B., Crosby, A. E., Davis, S., & Wilkins, N. (2017). *Preventing Suicide: A Technical Package of Policies, Programs, and Practices*. Atlanta, GA: National Center for Injury Prevention and Control, Centers for Disease Control and Prevention.

Townsend, W. (2010). Recovery services in rural settings, strengths and challenges influencing behavioral healthcare service delivery. *Rural Mental Health*, 34(1), 23–32.

US Department of Health and Human Services. (1999). Rockville, MD: *Substance Abuse and Mental Health Services Administration. Promising Practices*. Rockville, MD: Office of Rural Health Policy, Health Resources and Services Administration.

Vandiver, V. L. (2013). *Best Practices in Community Mental Health*. Chicago: Lyceum Books.

Weigel, D. (2009). *The Challenges of Rural Clinical Mental Health Counseling*. Weitz, Germany: VDM Verlag.

Whitaker, R. (2010). *Anatomy of an Epidemic*. New York: Broadway Books.

Wilson, W., Bangs, A., & Hatting, T. (February, 2015). *The Future of Rural Behavioral Health*. National Rural Health Association Policy Brief. www.ruralhealthnet.org

Wood, R. E. (2008). *Survival of Rural America: Small Victories and Bitter Harvests*. Lawrence: University Press of Kansas.

14 Suicide in Rural Areas

For over a decade, suicide rates in rural areas have surpassed urban rates. This chapter looks at the prevalence, causes, and risk factors inherent in suicide, the populations most at risk, and provides shocking statistics regarding suicide in America and its cost to our society. It investigates risk factors, prevention strategies, and treatment options, and concludes with a case study rooted in small town life.

Prevalence, Causes, and Risk Factors

Although most recent research studies indicate that the prevalence of mental health issues is generally similar in urban and rural areas, the exception to the rule is suicide. The suicide rates for both children and adults in rural areas are higher than their urban counterparts, a trend that has been consistent for more than a decade. The suicide rate is significantly higher among elderly males and Native American youth, and the rate of suicide appears to increase the more rural the population. While several factors have been suggested as contributing, in-depth analysis and research has not been conducted in multiple rural settings.

According to *Rural Mental Health* (Mohatt), individuals who live in rural areas frequently experience the "triple jeopardy" of being rural, poor, and uninsured. Compared to their urban counterparts, suicide attempts among individuals from rural areas are more frequently successful because their approaches are more likely to involve firearms and pesticides. Suicide makes up a major percentage of gun deaths in rural areas because there is an associated increased risk of suicide when a gun is owned. Firearm ownership is particularly high in rural areas because of their use in sports and hunting. Therefore, suicides in rural areas are more likely to be completed by rifles or shotguns than by handguns, which are more typically seen in urban areas. Self-poisoning is the most common method of suicide completion worldwide, and is largely a rural phenomenon. Approximately two-thirds of all pesticide poisonings are suicidal acts, resulting in 220,000 deaths annually worldwide. Refusal or avoidance of mental health services appears to be based to a large extent on a community's culture and has a dramatic impact on the increased occurrence of suicides in rural areas.

The scales of suicide completion between men and women weigh heavily on the side of men, who are four times as likely as women to commit suicide. This difference is similar in rural men both domestically and internationally, and it has been found that mental health deteriorates significantly as rurality increases. More rural young men than urban young men identify symptoms of depression, a leading risk factor for suicide. The Department of Health and Human Services estimates that approximately 20% of rural residents aged 55 and older have a mental disorder, and rural communities report significantly higher suicide rates than urban areas for both adults and children.

Some solutions include a drive to focus on preventive mental health care, reduce stigma associated with seeking mental health care, implement a school-based suicide-prevention curriculum, educate primary care providers, establish traditional and nontraditional suicide prevention/intervention programs, including telephone follow-up services, tele-mental health, crisis competency, computer-based telecommunications, traveling counselors, and more opportunities to avoid isolation such as social clubs and self-help groups. We are in dire need of additional solutions and much more research in order to increase suicide prevention.

Shocking Statistics About Suicide in America

Someone in the United States commits suicide every 13 minutes. That's 40,000 suicides annually. According to the Centers for Disease Control and Prevention (CDC), there were more than 41,000 suicides in America in 2013, and more than half of them were committed with a gun. Out of more than 33,000 gun deaths in 2013, almost two-thirds were gun suicides (Time Warner). According to *USA Today*, Americans are far more likely to kill themselves than each other. Homicides have fallen by half since 1991, but the suicide rate keeps climbing, making it the 10th leading cause of death and the second leading killer for those ages 15–34. The army suicide rate tripled from 2004 and 2012 as more than 2,000 GIs took their lives. Native Americans have the highest suicide rate in the country, at 1.8 times the national average.

Every suicide costs our society about $1 million in medical and lost-work expenses and emotionally victimizes an average of 10 other people. In *Thrive*, Layard and Clark report that as many people in the world die from suicide as from homicide and warfare combined. In 2000, over 815,000 people committed suicide, while 520,000 people were murdered, and 310,000 died as a result of war. In its 2014 article on the suicide crisis, *USA Today* argues that if we took suicide as seriously as we take AIDS or breast cancer, we could potentially save many lives as we have with our targeted focus on these other physical illnesses.

In 2015, the most recent figures available as of this writing, federal government statistics show that suicide was responsible for 44,193 deaths in the United States, which translates to about one suicide every 12 minutes. The same year, suicide ranked as the 10th leading cause of death and has been among the top 12 leading causes of death in America since 1975. Overall, suicide rates increased 28% between the years 2000 and 2015. It affects people throughout the lifespan. It is the third leading cause of death for children ages 10–14 years; the second leading cause of death among people aged 15–24; the fourth leading cause of death among people aged 25–44; the fifth leading cause among people aged 45–54; and the eighth leading cause among people aged 55–64.

The suicide rate is significantly higher among elderly males and Native American youth, and the rate of suicide appears to increase the more rural the population. While several factors have been suggested as contributing, in-depth analysis and research has not been conducted in multiple rural settings.

Many believe that the number of rural suicides is underreported. It is entirely possible that many rural deaths are attributed to farm-related accidents in order for a family living in a small town to save themselves from the shame that often accompanies survivors of the suicide of a loved one.

Suicides reflect only one facet of the problem. Substantially more people are hospitalized as a result of unsuccessful suicide attempts than are fatally injured, and an even greater number are either treated in hospital emergency rooms or are not treated at all. For example, during 2014, among adults aged 18 years and older, for every one suicide there were nine adults treated in hospital emergency departments for self-harm injuries, 27 who reported making a suicide attempt, and over 227 who reported seriously contemplating suicide.

Risk Factors and Prevention Strategies for Suicide

On the individual level, risk factors can include a history of depression or other mental illnesses, a prolonged sense of isolation and/or hopelessness, lack of social support, exposure to other suicides, substance abuse, victimization of abuse or violence, and genetic and biological factors.

An individual's relationships or lack of healthy relationships, and the quality of those relationships, such as whether or not they are conflict-laden or abusive as in domestic violence or emotional abuse, lack of social support and increased feeling of isolation, are all significant risk factors.

At the community and societal levels, geographic or social isolation, barriers to health care and lack of access to mental health providers and medications are risk factors that can be improved through involvement with civic groups, non-profit organizations, and local governments. More research is needed to determine if getting help via tele-therapy or calling hotlines or mobile crisis units are successful in reducing stigma, because a person does not have to go to a mental health clinic or practitioner's office.

Protective factors are the influences that buffer against the risk for suicide, and include effective coping and problem-solving skills, moral objections to suicide, strong and supportive relationships with others, connectedness to school and community, availability of quality and ongoing physical and mental health care, and reduced access to lethal means.

The available evidence from research suggests that strengthening economic supports may be one way to help buffer suicide risk. Studies that have examined historical suicidal trends have found that suicide rates increase during economic recessions marked by high unemployment rates, loss of jobs, and economic instability, and the rates decrease during stable economic times. No surprises there. But the information urges us to consider buffering these factors in order to keep suicide rates low or better yet, eradicate them altogether. Stone et al. suggest that strengthening economic support systems can help people stay in their homes or obtain affordable housing while also paying for necessities such as food and medical care, job training, and child care. Side benefits for our society would be reductions in foreclosure and eviction rates, increased family stability, and decreased rates of emotional distress and rates of suicide.

Treatment for Suicidal Individuals

Of course, the number one element of treatment and prevention for those who are suicidal is identifying ways to improve access to timely, affordable, quality mental health care. In rural areas, this is easier said than done, with the significant increase in travel time, shortage of mental health professionals, lack of insurance reimbursement, and the element of small town gossip for being seen entering a mental health clinic. Over 85 million Americans live in areas with an insufficient number of mental health providers, and this shortage is particularly severe among low-income communities, both urban and rural. According to Stone, research by Lang examined state mental health laws and suicide rates between 1990 and 2004 found that mental health parity laws, specifically, were associated with an approximate 5% reduction in suicide rates. This reduction, in the 29 states that had parity laws at that time, translated to the equivalent of 592 suicides *prevented*.

What else can be done to help prevent suicides? Changes to organizational culture through the implementation of supportive policies, for instance, can change social norms, encourage help-seeking, and demonstrate that good health and mental health are valued and that stigma and other risk factors for suicide are not. Modifying the characteristics of the physical environment to prevent harmful behavior such as access to lethal means can reduce suicide rates, particularly in times of crisis or transition. Safe practices and storage of medications, guns, knives, and other household items can reduce the risk of suicide by separating vulnerable people from easy access to lethal means. Guns should be locked in a secure place unloaded, with the ammunition locked up securely in a completely different location. Medicines can be kept in locked cabinets. Simple, commonsense measures such as these can have a profound effect in the prevention of suicide. Fear of asking someone if they are having suicidal thoughts remains high on the list of barriers to eliminating suicide.

Promoting connectedness among individuals and within communities through modeling peer norms and enhancing community engagement may protect against suicide. Peer norm programs seek to normalize factors for suicide such as seeking help, reaching out and talking with trusted adults, and promoting peer connectedness. These groups seek to shift group beliefs and promote positive social and behavioral changes. These kinds of approaches typically target youth and can be implemented through schools and community organizations.

Community engagement is an aspect of social capital. Examples include citizens participating in community clean-ups and other green activities, group sports, common interest groups, and the like in order to connect individuals to community members, organizations, and resources, which hopefully results in increased physical and mental health, reduced stress, and decreased depression, therefore reducing the risk of suicide.

Emotional literacy programs for children, parents, and families strengthen relationships while teaching coping and problem-solving skills. These programs focus on developing improved communication and coping skills while building resilience and stronger interpersonal bonds, which in turn help individuals make better choices for themselves. These programs can be implemented to all students in schools or can be done in small groups according to need. They can also be run by professionals in community settings. There is a huge need for parenting skills and family relationship programs, especially in rural areas, to provide caregivers with education and support. These programs are designed to improve parent–child relationships, help adults avoid parenting styles that have been dysfunctional for generations, and help children build better behavioral, emotional, and communication skills, as well as better awareness of their feelings and appropriate ways to express them. At present, there is a wide variety of programs available, including a program that encourages children to create and empower their own original superhero and then use it to learn about self-esteem, team-building, anti-bullying, and leadership skills.

Supporting vulnerable populations at risk for suicide remains the primary effort of suicide prevention. Effective response, crisis intervention, and evidence-based treatment, along with proactive systems for checking in with vulnerable people, are necessary. Communities should train teachers, coaches, emergency responders, and other community resources in how to respond effectively. Treatment can take the form of small groups or individual therapy, and the methods can include such evidence-based theoretical approaches as cognitive behavioral therapy (CBT), which has an offshoot called cognitive behavioral therapy for suicide prevention (CBT-SP), dialectical behavior therapy (DBT), Gestalt, narrative, and many others. The frequency of treatment, unfortunately, is partly determined by reimbursement policies. Many policies limit the number of visits to a mental health professional, while a few do not.

Recovery from suicidality varies greatly from person to person, and a mental health professional is the best person to determine frequency and duration of therapy sessions. When further therapy is not reimbursable, simple follow-up techniques such as sending postcards, phone calls, or letters can increase a client's sense of connectedness to a therapist and decrease feelings of isolation.

For families and loved ones of someone who has committed suicide, debriefing counseling and bereavement or support groups are highly recommended. They can go a long way toward healing, lessening survivor's guilt, feelings of depression, and complicated grief and trauma. It is also important at all levels of government to address gaps in responses, track progress of prevention efforts, and evaluate the impact of those efforts.

Rural Matters: The Last Straw

No emergency siren sounded at the fire hall. Police cars whizzed through town. The first one was at about 1 p.m., the second about 10 minutes later. I looked up from where I sat at my computer, took note, and got back to work thinking it could be about anything from a fire to a heart attack, stroke, or a traffic accident of some sort. Anything but what it was about: a young man, age 22, who committed suicide. He used a gun. It was fast and dirty. I found out when I went downtown and everyone already knew. No one knew the details yet, but everyone looked shocked. He spent his whole life in this town, was known by almost everyone and remembered fondly as a quiet, nice kid. He lost his way after high school and became addicted to drugs, they told each other. I knew him well enough, but in a very different way.

I got a call from his mother early last summer asking me if he could come to me for therapy. He was using heroin and had been for some time. I didn't know him except by name. We talked for a while and then scheduled an appointment. When Wayne arrived, he looked sober and alert. He said he'd been off drugs for 6 days. He was a soft-spoken kind of guy, but surprised me by talking about himself quite a bit. I asked questions here and there, but he did most of the talking. I began to get to know him in an emotionally intimate way.

I continued to see him twice a week for most of the summer. He also had a counselor at the county drug and alcohol clinic. He shared with me things he was thinking and feeling about drugs, women, work, family, and his future. He had a trade as a mechanic and enjoyed his work for the most part. He really enjoyed fixing up old cars; talking about it brought a sparkle to his dark eyes. Those eyes were a deep brown, almost black, almost impenetrable. He continued to stay clean as far as I could tell, and was just starting to feel better about himself when he suddenly stopped coming. I tried phoning him several times with no response. I didn't run into him around town, which is surprising given the size of our town.

I was stunned when I heard the news. I stared in disbelief picturing his youthful face in my mind as clear as if he were right in front of me. This was the sixth suicide in Delaware County in 2 months. The others occurred at

Vandiver, V. L. (2013). *Best Practices in Community Mental Health*. Chicago: Lyceum Books.

Weigel, D. (2009). *The Challenges of Rural Clinical Mental Health Counseling*. Weitz, Germany: VDM Verlag.

Whitaker, R. (2010). *Anatomy of an Epidemic*. New York: Broadway Books.

Wood, R. E. (2008). *Survival of Rural America: Small Victories and Bitter Harvests*. Lawrence: University Press of Kansas.

15 A Day in the Life of a Rural Mental Health Practitioner

This chapter lays out a day in the life of a rural mental health practitioner, including a typical ride to work and coping with the rural landscape, dealing with professional isolation and other occupational hazards, limitations placed on rural practitioners, the ins and outs of running a rural private practice, and a case study.

Occupational Hazards

Many are the occupational hazards of the rural mental health practitioner. Coping with the rural environment is not to be underestimated. Mother Nature rules in this domain, and winters can be long and harsh. All it takes is a dusting of snow to make the roads slippery, and the weather can and does turn on a dime. The locals will tell you if you don't like the weather here, wait 10 minutes. I've experienced it enough to know that it is true. Summers are usually beautiful but not without severe thunderstorms, hailstorms, sizzling hot weeks of full humidity and even an occasional frost in July (I've heard there was once one in August, but I haven't experienced it myself).

Professional isolation is one occupational hazard I was not prepared for. It is not easy to form close friendships with people when you are working therapeutically with either them or their family members. It is common for many rural practitioners to have their closest friends living outside their communities. There have been several times when I was concerned that someone would act vindictively toward myself or a family member. The first time was when I called the state child abuse hotline about a child who stated that his father whipped him with a belt. My concern arose because there were a limited number of people with whom the child interacted. Although the hotline calls are confidential, if the child's father figured out it was me who called, and he now has an open Child Protective Services case against him, his anger might cause him to do even more harm.

Once the mother of a child I worked with showed up at my house on a Saturday evening feeling suicidal. I felt I couldn't turn her away, so I phoned the state police who promptly showed up at my house. The trooper was going to take her to a crisis center an hour and a half away. I argued with him that she had recently been at the crisis center an hour away in the opposite direction and that he should take her there because they had her records and were familiar with her. His response was that he was mandated to take anyone from this town and northward to the center an hour and a half away. I pleaded again. After conferring by phone with his higher-ups outside on my freezing cold porch, he came in with a solution. He would drive her to the nearby hospital, 12 miles away, which was designated a Critical Access Hospital, and from there the hospital could send her the remaining 45 minutes to the center she had been at. That is what ultimately happened, and family members took care of the kids. The crisis center kept her for several weeks. It was the first time I had state troopers at my house, and hopefully the last.

Yet another occupational hazard is the difficulty of establishing firm boundaries between work time and off time. So while I was very visible in town events as a volunteer my first years of living here, I have had to somewhat limit what I give back to the community because it is difficult for people dealing with issues important to them to save them for a regular appointment. This issue is by no means limited to mental health professionals; it is also common to lawyers, doctors, teachers, plumbers, and contractors. Once I lived here for a few years, almost everyone I encountered when I walked to the store, or walked my dog, is a client, or the family member of a client, or someone who wants to talk about my work.

Another unexpected outcome of becoming a private mental health practitioner in a rural area is that is better to be a generalist. I see mainly children, but I also work with adolescents, adults, couples, and families. In order to serve the needs of the community, not only must I see clients in all phases of the human lifespan, but I need many theoretical tools in my toolbox because there is no one-size-fits-all theory. While some people don't mind going back to their childhoods in great detail, others find these "depth psychologies" to be unnecessarily regressive and too long term for their liking. I need to have other theoretical models and techniques in my repertoire, in order to use them as needed for different people in different situations. Some therapeutic methods such as CBT (cognitive behavioral therapy) and DBT (dialectical behavioral therapy) are suited for some age groups through the lifespan but can be detrimental to other age groups.

I recently heard about an organization called the Delaware County Rural Healthcare Alliance. I was excited and wondered if I could attend a committee meeting and perhaps join as a regular member. I called to ask if they dealt with any mental health issues and was shocked to hear the answer was no. The Alliance focuses on many wonderful things for the county, including chronic disease prevention, maternal and newborn health, disaster preparedness, nutrition education, and so forth. Is mental health not an important enough part of overall health to include in a health care committee?

Another occupational hazard for rural practitioners was the subject of a study in the *Journal of Rural Community Psychology* (Kos and DeStefano). The study found that mental health practitioners progress through professional burnout in a sequence of internal processes. First comes emotional exhaustion, arising in response to the demands of the work environment. This changes to depersonalization as clinicians try to distance themselves from clients in order to conserve their own psychic energy and as a coping mechanism in order to deal with exhaustion. The combination of exhaustion and an impoverished relationship with clients causes a sense of diminished personal efficacy as the work loses its meaning. Lack of personal accomplishment fans the flames of the above process. Group supervision, rather than strictly individual supervision, might create more of a sense of community among practitioners as well as encourage brainstorming for better solutions to work issues. Providing opportunities for professional and personal development to offset the feeling of isolation from colleagues is also a commonsense best practice.

My Ride to Work

My ride to work is an hour long in good weather. It brings me diagonally across the county from the northeastern corner to near the southwestern corner. The ride consists of one traffic light (which could be avoided if I really wanted to), two one-lane bridges, three hairpin curves in the road, one of which is on a steep slope, over a dozen dairy farms, vacant fields, steep mountain slopes, rivers that sometimes overflow, a maple syrup enterprise, many flocks of sheep, goats, cows of different kinds, and a horse rehabilitation center. The sky never looks the same on the ride to and from, with it overcast and dark at times, at other times pure sunshine on the fields of corn and grain, and frequently in the winter, miles of sparkling snow and ice.

I pass several tipping silos, deserted barns, bits of unpaved road, and mud patches (which, by the way, are as slippery as ice), and many are the ruts in the road. Many days there are trucks loaded with lumber coming at me from the opposite direction, and hay wagons brimming with rectangular bales (most use the large circular bales, which weigh 800 pounds are harder to transport). Frequently on the roads are trucks transporting livestock: chickens, cows, pigs, lambs, goats, and even horses. They weigh heavily on the one-lane bridges that cross the rivers at various intervals. I pass two covered wooden bridges and sometimes cross one just for effect. I pass many school buses that collect children on the backroads and drive them to the nearest central school, which could take an hour or more.

What I don't see are windmills for green energy, more creameries to process milk, more supermarkets, movie theaters, and medical clinics. These are spread much further apart from each other and require a car to reach. At least in my area, I don't see much in the way of any kind of economic development. I do see many people packing it in and moving to areas with more opportunity economically, educationally, medically and in just about any area of needed services.

My Decision to Enter Private Practice

For me, the decision to start a private practice was not a direct one. After years of working at various agencies and facilities for low pay, the decision to go out on my own limb and test the private practice waters was to a large extent economic. In a rural area where there are few jobs to be had, it makes sense to take a leap of faith and create your own job—or patch several part-time jobs together, because it's easier to get an hourly job with no benefits than to get a full-time job with salary and benefits, especially with no license parity. The clinic where I'm the coordinator for the Single Point of Access (SPOA) program needs a clinician, but they are not allowed by the state Office of Mental Health to consider hiring me for that position regardless of the fact that I have a state issued license.

I have always been a hard worker, so I wasn't worried about working for myself from that perspective. I experienced firsthand the phenomenon of representing two different roles in the community and the need to respect confidentiality. What I did worry about was community acceptance, because I am not a native to the area. Practitioners cannot just move to the country, hang out a shingle, and expect to be flooded with clients. Anyone wishing to do this must first and foremost be an accepted community member. They must be seen as credible by the community at large, and this does not happen quickly. Those of us who are transplants need to become involved with the community and its people on a personal basis, which involves volunteering for various organizations and causes in the area, joining organizational boards of directors. To my benefit, however, when I did these things over a period of several years, I learned how things really happen in my community, who to call for what, and what to call whom. I also learned who is related to who, and plenty of background stories and gossip, obviously unsolicited.

When dealing with community and personal interactions, no one in a rural area has personal privacy. Rural practitioners must develop ways to cope with these situations in order to continue to live and practice in the same small town. It's a lot like walking a tightrope.

When it comes to running and managing a rural private mental health practice, I have several clients who live in the area with no car or driver's license, whether revoked or never received. Therefore I decided it was necessary, in order to serve the native local population, to make home visits. I set limits for the visits in terms of accessibility, not wanting to travel muddy dirt roads or icy back roads in the winter. Most of those who needed me to make home visits live in accessible areas.

It is of the utmost importance to decode and begin to live within the prevailing rural ethic. That includes not only ethics, but also politics, attitudes about diversity, religion, professional and educational status, socioeconomic status, and lifestyle choices. It also includes some lesser topics such as educational attitudes, sports abilities and interests, willingness to volunteer for various things, ability to get to know everyone's automobile and waving whenever we pass them on the road. Also important is the degree of self-reliance you run your life with. Already struggling with limited resources by definition, rural populations have all they can do to gather the resources necessary to help their own. To make a generalization, it has been my experience that the rural population admires those who keep worries to themselves and take care of their own lives. Gossip is the kiss of death in rural social life. While gossiping might initially make you some friends, very soon no one will trust you because of it. In rural areas, comfort within the therapist/client relationship is determined foremost by the level of trust in the confidentiality factor. While mental health practitioners are trained to think in terms of ambiguity, rural folks have little tolerance for it, wanting straightforward answers. And while mental health professionals by definition believe in the possibility and desirability of change, rural populations often doubt that changes can be made.

Rural practice forces one to be creative, to improvise, to always have a Plan B, and to grow stronger and more self-reliant. I have had the absolute best of times of my life here and also the absolute worst. My concern for my clients is genuine and they know it. Although it has not been easy, I have grown incredibly as a professional, probably much more so because I took the leap and went into private practice. I know I have helped many individuals and families, prevented some tragedies, acted as mentor and role model, and made some mistakes as well. Hopefully I have brought peace to some. You know a place is your true home when it starts to break your heart, when you begin to worry about the fate of the land, both in terms of ecology and future development; when you know the shorthand of who is related to who and some family history about many families who make up the fabric of community; when the community comes to your aid with dinners, rides, and cards from people you never met when you go through cancer treatment; when you have no desire to be anywhere else, because, after all, this is your adopted home where your heart lives.

The wearing of many hats is a commonly accepted and even expected phenomenon. People in my town know me as a counselor (I feel the word counselor has less stigma than the word "therapist"). They also know me as a wife, mother, dog owner, and probably several other labels I'd rather not know.

I have been invited to parties and gatherings in which I knew clients would be attending. In my initial appointments with people, I address the possibility of meeting outside the office by suggesting that, if they agree, if I ever run into them elsewhere, I will give them a friendly hello and keep walking, but no one will know how we know each other. In small town life it is commonplace to know many people, at least enough to give a sincere hello. So far, everyone has been fine with it, and this tactic has worked well. I have worked with children who were in my daughter's class on several occasions, making sure they understood that I will never let anyone know of our arrangement, but they are free to let others know if they so desire. One of these kids in particular came to work with me during a difficult time in her life. We worked together on a short-term basis. The following year she worked under me at one of my jobs, making me her boss. I hope that in both facets of our relationship, I was a good mentor to her. I know I learned from her struggles. She has grown immensely as a person and I miss her now that she being has gone off to college.

Rural Matters: A Paper Person

It's another picture-perfect day in the Catskills. Thick fog sank into the valleys last night like wet cotton balls, and the fall leaves darkened two shades. When the fog burns off, the sky will be a brilliant blue with the sun shining in triumph.

I leave for work at 8 a.m. sharp, needing to be there by 9 a.m. How many times do my ears pop as I ascend the more than 3,000-foot mountain road and back down again? The road wound tight as a coil slows me down, but not as much as the hay wagon I am stuck behind. Spraying flecks of hay as it clunks down the mountain, I can't go any slower if I try. I worry I'll be late for a meeting.

When I finally arrive, I don't have time to make coffee. I turn my computer on, check messages, and make notes to begin the work day. I now have a purely administrative job, housed in the children's Community Mental Health Clinic. I am not allowed to practice as a therapist here because the state does not recognize my license with parity, in spite of the fact that they set up the requirements and issued the license. So, here I am, happy to be here in this environment where I feel comfortable to be learning a macro version of the mental health care system. My job is to work with difficult cases and hook them up to services by way of a monthly committee meeting that representatives from various agencies attend and help determine which services are appropriate for each case.

I listen to my messages and am startled to learn that one of them, from the county Department of Social Services, is asking me to return the call, and it's about none other than Nicki. When we connect, she tells me that there is an urgent need for more services for Nicki now that she is no longer in her prospective adoptive home, but is back at the agency-operated foster care home. She wants to have this case reviewed by my program's committee at the next meeting. I fill her in on the procedures and the paperwork she needs to submit, and we end the phone call.

In this job, I refer to the files that are submitted for review as "paper people." I rarely have a visual of the child to match to the name, no voice, no sense of personality. I only have a mental health diagnosis if there is one, and a psychosocial review by the therapist. Sometimes the names blend together in my mind. I wish we could require a photograph with each application so they would have another dimension in my mind. Nevertheless, to see Nicki's name on an application to the program at this job, having been so involved with her case for a year and a half is just so strange. I feel uneasy about it.

The application comes by fax the following day and I review it with the same eye as I do all the applications, thinking through finding the best match of services for this particular case. I see her brilliant blue eyes, I hear her voice and see her wry smile, and I'm reminded of her strengths. But this system is not a one that focuses on strengths. It doesn't matter that she has a high IQ for her 7 years of age, that she can charm a coin from anyone's hand if she so desires. No, the committee and I hear about her weaknesses, or "deficits" as they're sometimes called.

I wonder if she misses me or ever thinks about me. I wonder if she remembers the many things I worked with her on, tried to teach her. I wonder if she felt my nonjudgmental stance, if she felt my love. I remember the time she nearly trashed my office, throwing things, nearly breaking windows, as she raged and vented. I often refer to this stage as "the purge." And although it is necessary, I worried she would not be able to stop, but she did. And then she sank to the floor and sobbed. I sat next to her, my hand gently on her back, whispering to her, "it's OK, you're going to be alright. Go ahead and cry as long as you need to."

So, what's happened between then and now in Nicki's life? Her conduct is a combination of pathological and behavioral, like apples and oranges in a cornucopia of emotion. There is no uniform plan for reacting to her behavior between her teachers, her foster home, her after-school care, her therapist, and her prospective adoptive family. No teamwork, no coordination. Her medications have been changed several times, with no more than a few weeks' improvement. I recommended a residential evaluation for her over a year ago, but my solicited advice was ignored. She is now in danger of being placed in a long-term residential treatment facility at 7 years of age.

Her beautiful little face comes to mind, and I feel we've all failed her. That day we sat on the floor in my office, she sobbed for a long, long time as daylight slowly faded. At the end, she stood up and extended her hand to help me stand. In that moment, she pulled me completely into her pain, a pain so deep and large I don't know how she can manage it. Her Teddy bear dangled from her other hand, so vulnerable and raw in its complete baldness.

References

Bagalman, E. (2016). *The Helping Families in Mental Health Crisis Reform Act of 2016*. Washington, DC: Congressional Research Service.

Bailey, C., Jensen, L., & Ransom, E. (2014). *Rural America in a Globalizing World*. Morgantown: West Virginia University Press.

Bain, S. F. (November, 2010). Itinerant counseling services for rural communities: A win/win opportunity. *Journal of Rural Community Psychology*, E13(1).

Berg-Cross, L., Reviere, R., Miller, J., Chappell, A., & Salmon, A. (2001). Certification of mental health advocates: A call to action. *Journal of Rural Community Psychology*, E14(1).

Bird, D. C., Dempsey, P., & Hartley, D. (2001). *Efforts to Address Mental Health Workforce Needs in Underserved Rural Areas*. University of Southern Maine, Institute for Health Policy, Maine Rural Health Research Center (Working Paper #23).

Carter, R. (2010). *Within Our Reach: Ending the Mental Health Crisis*. Emmaus, PA: Rodale Books.

Castle, E. (Ed.). (1995). *The Changing American Countryside: Rural People and Places*. Lawrence: University Press of Kansas.

Centers for Disease Control and Prevention (CDC). (December 18, 2015). Increases in Drug and Opioid Overdose Deaths—United States, 2000–2014. *Morbidity and Mortality Weekly Report*, 64(50), 1378–1382.

Cloke, P., Marsden, T., & Mooney, P. H. (Eds.). (2006). *Handbook of Rural Studies*. Thousand Oaks, CA: Sage.

Coalition for Mental Health Reform. (July 6, 2016). *Concerns With the Helping Families in Mental Health: Crisis Act of 2015—Passed in the House of Representatives*.

Cornell University. (2010). *Poverty, Local and Regional Government, Energy, Economic and Workforce Development, Agriculture and Food Systems*. Ithaca, NY. www.cornell.edu.

Davidson, O. G. (1996). *Broken Heartland: The Rise of America's Rural Ghetto*. Iowa City: University of Iowa Press.

Gladding, S. T. (1997). *Community and Agency Counseling*. Upper Saddle River, NJ: Prentice-Hall.

Goldman, H. H., Buck, J. A., & Thompson, K. S. (2009). *Transforming Mental Health Services: Implementing the Federal Agenda for Change*. Arlington, VA: American Psychiatric Association.

Grantham, D. (February 1, 2017). *The Challenge of Affordable Health Care: The ACA and Beyond*. Washington, DC: National Association of County Behavioral Health and Developmental Disability Directors.

Hartley. D., Bird, D., Lambert, D., & Coffin, J. (November, 2002). *The Role of Community Mental Health Centers as Rural Safety Net Providers*. Portland: University of Southern Maine, Edmund S. Muskie School of Public Service, Maine Rural Health Research Center (Working Paper #30).

Hartley, D., Ziller, E., Lambert, D., Loux, S., & Bird, D. (October, 2002). *State Licensure Laws and the Mental Health Professions: Implications For the Rural Mental Health Workforce*. Portland: University of Southern Maine, Edmund S. Muskie School of Public Service, Maine Rural Health Research Center (Working Paper #29).

Hill, M. (1997). *Diary of a Country Therapist*. New York: Haworth Press.

Imig, A. (July 12, 2016). Small But Mighty: Perspectives of Rural Mental Health Counselors. *The Professional Counselor*. www.nbcc.org.

Kennedy Forum. (2016). *Navigating the New Frontier of Mental Health and Addiction: A Guide for the 115th Congress*. www.parityregistry.org; www.thekennedyforum.org; www.paritytrack.org.

Kennedy, P. J. (2015). *A Common Struggle: A Personal Journey Through the Past and Future of Mental Illness and Addiction*. New York: Blue Rider Press.

Kos, M. E., & DeStefano, T. J. (2000). The investigation of the developmental course of Burnout among rural clinicians. *Journal of Rural Community Psychology*, E14(1).

Lightburn, A., & Sessions, P. (2006). *Handbook of Community-Based Clinical Practice*. New York: Oxford University Press.

Manderscheid, R. (March 23, 2015). *Stigma Kills: On the Five "P's" of Inclusion and Social Justice*. www.nacbhdd.org.

Manderscheid, R. (June 7, 2016). Helping rural counties keep abreast of urban counterparts. *Behavioral Healthcare Magazine.* www.behavioral.net.

Mohatt, D. F. (2016). *Rural Mental Health: Challenges and Opportunities Caring for the Country.* Boulder, CO: Western Interstate Commission for Higher Education.

Morris, J. (2009, Summer). Marriage and family therapists expand access to mental health services in rural areas. *Journal of Rural Community Psychology*, E12(1).

Morris, J.A. (1997). *Practicing Psychology in Rural Settings.* Washington, DC: American Psychological Association.

National Rural Health Association, Government Affairs Office (October, 2008). *Policy Position: Workforce Series—Rural Behavioral Health.* Washington, DC.

New Freedom Commission on Mental Health (2003). *Achieving the Promise: Transforming Mental Health Care in America.* Final. DHHS Pub. Co. SMA-03-3832. Rockville, MD.

Perry, M. (2002). *Population: 485, Meeting Your Neighbors One Siren at a Time.* New York: Harper Perennial.

Quinn, M. (September, 2016). *Rural America Finally Gets Mental Health Help.* www.governing.com/templates.gov_print_article.

Ranier, J.P. (2010). The road much less traveled: Treating rural and isolated clients. *Journal of Clinical Psychology: In Session*, 66(5), 475–478.

Rhodes, P. (Ed.). (2014). *Mental Health and Rural America.* New York: Nova Science.

Robert, D. (Ed.). (1992). *Psychological Practice in Small Towns and Rural Areas.* Binghamton, NY: Haworth Press.

Rural Policy Research Institute. (2016). www.rupri.org.

Sawyer, D., Gale, J., & Lambert, D. (2006). *Rural and Frontier Mental and Behavioral Health Care: Barriers, Effective Policy Strategies, and Best Practices.* Washington, DC: National Association for Rural Mental Health.

Schank, J., & Skovholt, T. (2006). *Ethical Practice in Small Communities: Challenges and Rewards for Psychologists.* Washington, DC: American Psychological Association.

Smalley, K.B., Warren, J., & Rainer, J. (Eds.). (2012). *Rural Mental Health: Issues, Policies, and Best Practices.* New York: Springer.

Smalley, K.B., Yancey, C.T., Warren, J.C., Naufel, K., Ryan, R., & Pugh, J.L. (2010). Rural mental health and psychological treatment: A review for practitioners. *Journal of Clinical Psychology: In Session*, 66(5), 479–489.

Smith, A. (2003). Rural mental health counseling: One example of practicing what the research preaches. *Journal of Rural Community Psychology*, E6(2), Fall.

Stamm, B.H. (Ed.). (2003). *Rural Behavioral Health Care.* Washington, DC: American Psychological Association.

Vandiver, V.L. (2012). *Best Practices in Community Mental Health.* Chicago: Lyceum Books.

Weigel, D. (2009). *The Challenges of Rural Clinical Mental Health Counseling.* Weitz, Germany: VDM Verlag.

Wood, R.E. (2008). *Survival of Rural America: Small Victories and Bitter Harvests.* Lawrence: University Press of Kansas.

Ziller, E. (2002). *State Licensure Laws and the Mental Health Professions: Implications for the Rural Mental Health Workforce.* Portland, ME: Cutler Institute for Health and Social Policy.

16 The Rural Economy in Transition

The rural economy is in constant transition out of necessity. Rural areas have always had to keep redefining themselves. This chapter surveys the history of America's rural economy and the mental health toll this all takes on individuals, families, and the community. It also looks at the economic side of the farm crisis, the effect of changes in agricultural technology, and suggestions to consider for the future of rural economies.

Redefining Livelihood

In this early part of the 21st century, the rural economy remains in transition. The percentage of people making their livelihood from farming is down to 1.9% and is continuing to drop. The skiing, hunting, fishing, post-9/11 influx, vacationing, and second home owners are holding up the local economy these days, and some years it is a more difficult struggle than others. According to Thomas in *Critical Rural Theory*, convenience stores attached to gas stations are found in 124 towns in the region, while supermarkets are found in only 44 of them. I have to drive at least 12 miles in either direction, one way, to find a supermarket. According to a 2005 study of supermarket prices in the region, prices were lower in the largest and most prosperous markets, meaning that residents of smaller communities (which tend to be those with the highest poverty rates and lowest education rates) are paying more for food and basic supplies.

There are some areas of significant hope for these areas with the development of the alternative fuels industry and wind power, the trend toward buying and eating locally grown foods, niche farms, ecological sustainability, the advancements in technology and internet capability, growth in the numbers of rural entrepreneurs, and the desire of a growing number of people to lead a simpler life, one that is more in tune with nature. This phenomenon was highly apparent in the years following 9/11, when so many rural towns experienced a noticeable flurry of urbanites relocating here where they felt safer. Many told me that their children developed asthma in the months following that national catastrophe, and that they believed the clean country air would be healing to them. We hadn't seen that level of influx since the Back to the Land movement in the 1980s. Whether or not many of them remained here for the long term is not documented.

In the year 1790, farmers made up 90% of the workforce in the United States. In 1900, at the turn of the previous century, most Americans lived in rural communities, with farmers accounting for almost 40% of the US workforce. In 1800, only 2% of the planet's population lived in cities. By 1900 that number was 12%, and by 2000 it was over 47%. In 2008 the urban population of the planet outnumbered the rural population for the first time ever (Wood, p. 4). Most rural communities reached their population peak between 1900 and 1950, before the interstate highway system was built and before large-scale industrialized farming began. Industrialized farming allows us to yield about three times as much food on one-third of the land and using two-thirds of the manpower as we used prior to World War II. That trend is fully expected to continue, eliminating many farm-related jobs.

For the first half of the 20th century, much of the area's economy was based on tourism, with large-scale hotels bustling with people from New York City spending their summers in the country air. Most of those hotels are no longer standing, but they were imposing structures on a grand scale, and they were well known. Many tuberculosis sufferers came to the area to breathe the fresh air with hope to heal. Eventually the hotel culture became known for its family-style accommodations and comedy acts. It was known as the Borscht Belt after its largely Jewish customers during the 1950s and 1960s. The movie *Dirty Dancing* is about this era in the grand hotels and resorts of the Catskill Mountains.

Currently in America, the poorest rural areas are in Appalachia, the East, and the South. These are areas in decay, the decline of which began when the population began to migrate in larger numbers to urban areas. It began when highways and rail lines bypassed the town or stopped traveling through the area. Roxbury is a prime example of a once thriving town that was bypassed by larger highways, and whose rail tracks are now walking and biking paths. There were two gas stations in town, one owned by my husband's family. There was a small grocery shop, hardware store, butcher shop, pharmacy, and a movie theater. Most were gone before I arrived 25 years ago, and not one of these exists in town now and hasn't in more than a decade.

In *The Other America*, Michael Harrington writes of the dilemma displaced farmers and miners have in rural America. The unemployed men who were displaced from the mines and farms have themselves become surplus commodities. A place without its young is a place without hope. The Appalachian population as well as that of the rural poor all over America are the workings of a curious inverse relationship, namely that a technological revolution in agriculture created the conditions for the persistence of poverty. One cannot raise the echelons of society without benefiting everyone from the bottom up. Harrington concludes that the most distinguishing mark of the other America is its communal sense of hopelessness.

One potential solution is for colleges and universities teaching rural health and mental health to require students to do rural internships. Research has shown the likelihood that the prolonged exposure to rurality increases the likelihood that more graduates will choose to practice in a rural setting.

Another trend to boost the economy in rural areas is to make them tourist destinations. In my area, the wedding "industry" has brought hundreds of people to the area each weekend of the summer. These guests need everything while they are here, from food to lodging, flowers, gasoline, hair stylists, makeup artists, parking, and charter bus transportation. It has proved to be a boost to our otherwise lagging economy. Rural counties can turn historical buildings into tourist designations, coordinate art studio tours and historic building tours, and can turn protected federal and state land into monitored recreation centers. Farm-to-table meals are popular ways to attract tourists, as are festivals of different kinds. There are many opportunities for hiking, wildflower and bird walks, food foraging hikes, snowmobiling, skiing, bicycling, skating, hunting, boating, leaf-peeping, and so much more.

In the 1970s, anthropologist Walter Goldschmidt added to the growing debate about agriculture and its structure. His classic study, *As You Sow*, compared two communities of similar size. The first one had an agricultural system composed largely of mid-sized owner-operators and the other of large, absentee-owned farms. His findings were severely in contrast. The small farm community supported nearly twice as many businesses as the industrial farm community and two-thirds more retail trade. In the small farm community, there were 20% more people per dollar of crop sales, and half the breadwinners were self-employed. Two-thirds of the people in the industrial farm were hourly wage laborers, with less than one-fifth of paid workers being self-employed. The small farm community had four elementary schools and a high school while the industrial farm community had only one elementary school. The small farm community had three parks and two newspapers, while the industrial farm community had only one corporate-owned playground and one newspaper. Additionally, the small farm community had twice the number of civic organizations and churches.

The American Agriculture Movement (AAM) perhaps most clearly manifests the values of family-oriented farming. This national organization bills itself as the voice of the family farmer and explicitly positions itself against industrial interests. It took the formation of the AAM and its public protests in 1977–1979 to galvanize public interest in the issue of structure. According to the organization, the AAM was born out of desperation in 1977 after Congress enacted a farm bill that guaranteed 4 more years of payments to farmers below their production costs.

In 1981, the US Department of Agriculture put out a report that legitimized the question of who benefits from agricultural policy and government farm programs, a question with immense political and policy consequences that had gone largely unexamined. Among the conclusions of the report were that tax policy is biased toward larger farms and wealthy investors, and the marketing system has increasingly oriented itself to serving larger producers.

Commodity price support programs and credit services have benefited larger producers and landlords. The report concluded that there is little or no efficiency to be gained from the further expansion of large farms because as farms continue to grow larger, additional labor is required, and where is that minimum wage migrant working type of help going to come from anyway? It creates the opposite of a healthy, balanced economy in the agricultural industry.

There are several schools of thought regarding agricultural policy and family farmers. One view is that of the University of California Davis Small Farm Program, which believes that,

> In many rural communities, family scale farms provide an economic foundation, generating revenues, taxes, and jobs for local communities . . . Small farms are perceived by the commission as providing healthy environments to raise families. Smaller family scale operations contribute to greater diversity in agricultural diversity of ownership, cropping systems, biological organization, cultures and traditions. And, reiterating the Jeffersonian perspective, the commission noted that landowners who rely on local businesses and services for their needs are more likely to have a stake in the well-being of the community.

A second viewpoint is espoused by the AAM and other farm activists groups that organized in the 1970s and 1980s. Their primary concern is with saving the farm family. They understand family farming as a tradition that is worth preserving. To that end, they advocate for commodity price supports to guarantee that these operations will be able to survive. Perhaps the greatest achievement of the AAM, through its engagement with government and advocacy for mid-sized family farms, has been to bring the question of structure and relative policy benefits to the foreground.

It should not be a political act to go to the supermarket, but it has become that for me. I wander the aisles wondering if this product was grown locally. I wonder what the carbon footprint is on the production and transportation of the product. I wonder if the organic produce I'm buying is truly organic, and I hope the land is being treated in a sustainable way. I wonder if the product I am buying was produced by someone who was treated fairly and earned a living wage.

The AAM has been a powerful resource, especially for men, because it has helped them find a language enabling them to admit to feeling loss, frustration, and vulnerability. They shared their stories, and in doing so, they could see that their experiences and their feelings were similar. It helped reduce stigma and level the emotional playing field. Hopefully the sharing of feelings will provide reason to consider the kind of future we want to have and the meaning of human advancement. And hopefully, this will yield the emotional power required to move us to the kind of future that has greater social justice and parity for everyone.

For people who did give up their farms after a long struggle, the final reality is often remembered as the days the cows left and the barn was empty.

I watched helplessly as a woman farmer gave up her four dozen Holstein cows one particularly bleak spring. They were loaded onto several tractor trailers and taken to a farm in West Virginia. She watched, her hands covering the tears streaming down her face as she walked slowly into the farmhouse and closed the door on the scene.

According to Fitchen in *Endangered Spaces, Enduring Places*, because farm families in financial danger did not turn to one another, they certainly were not going to turn to services such as welfare or Medicaid for help. Many hard-hit farm families would have been ineligible for the usual assistance programs because of their farm assets; nevertheless, their pride kept them from seeking what they considered to be government handouts to the poor. They preferred to get through on their own, from their own friends and families for things such as loans of equipment or cows, or a lower rental charge for land. For farmers, their herd is tied up in their identity, their pride, and their status in the farming community. So many of them showed calves at the county fair when they were youngsters, and this lifestyle is an extension of that. Their love for their herds runs very deep. To many, the highest compliment they can receive is that they are a good cow family.

In Delaware County and the surrounding area, local extension agents estimated that about one-third of farmers were not in serious trouble during the 1980s. In fact, some farm operations weathered the decade reasonably well and a few quite profitably, although not without some strain. In addition to the dairy industry, the area was well known for growing mass quantities of cauliflower.

Inevitably, changes in agriculture affect the formal organizational life of rural communities, but this is not specifically due to the farm crisis. Failing small independent farming communities experienced a cultural crisis because of the change from farming community to non-farming community, a change not easily reversible.

Rural populations need to learn to think in an open-minded way, not settling for that "we've never done it that way before" kind of mentality. We need to encourage the development of alternative biofuels such as grass/hay pellets, which maintain productive open space and create new job opportunities. We also must shed that "not in my backyard" kind of thinking and be open enough to encourage the production of wind power, methane gas, ethanol, hydro and solar energy development, and investigate cryogenic fuels such as liquid hydrogen, coal gasification, geothermal energy, and the use of waste tires for oil. And more than anything, we need more research on the cost-effectiveness and feasibility of growing these alternative energy systems. Developing renewable energy systems, or "greening up," can not only enhance the prosperity of rural agricultural communities, but it might just be the thing that saves them.

In the Catskill Mountains where I live, for instance, the construction of water reservoirs and tunnels over a 150-year period for the benefit of New York City has resulted in a landscape of large forested preserves surrounding the reservoirs and an agricultural landscape at a distance from the water supply. This landscape is considered "natural" in that it is devoid of people, but they are forgetting the inhabitants who have lived here for thousands of years. It's as if "nature" has been defined as land without people. The cultural definition is supported by the fact that New York City no longer needs this portion of its hinterland for rural production, as such products are acquired from further afield—in a sense the "world" is New York's hinterland—enabling urban elites to pursue policies that limit this function of the Catskills. In this case, water is the primary motivator to preserve the Catskills. Through preservation the city has been able to keep its water supply pure enough to avoid an order by the Environmental Protection Agency to build a costly filtration system. The vast lands held by New York City are now opened to hikers, boaters, and hunters for recreational purposes. The sad rural truth is that the area and its inhabitants are stripped of self-determination, and the importance of urban needs is assumed to be greater than rural interests. This is urbanormativity at its best.

Here are some astounding statistics: in 1790, farmers made up approximately 90% of America's workforce. By 1900, the percentage of farmers had dwindled down to about 40%, and by 2000, that number shrank to 1.9%. According to Wood, currently, one farmer produces more than five farmers did in 1940, and the number of farmers in the country has dropped almost 80% from 14 million in 1910 to about three million today. In addition, the number of farms has plummeted, from over six million in 1910 to about two million today. When one farmer is forced to leave a community, there is an economic loss estimated at $72,000.

Because of their proximity to agricultural crops, rural people run a greater risk of developing cancer from exposure to pesticides than do consumers in general. This can be true both if the farms are actively using pesticides, or if the pesticides are left in the ground from former use. The problem of groundwater contamination from farm chemicals is especially serious in rural America, where 97% of the population depends on underground aquifers for its water supply. Groundwater studies in rural areas have yielded sobering results, with dozens of pesticides found in it. The single most shocking development in agriculture is the recent discovery of cancer hot spots, which are rural communities in which cancer rates zoom far above a normal range.

"In a world short on fossil fuels or any viable replacement for them," writes Wood in the Survival of Rural America,

> the necessity of "resettling the countryside"—to gather dispersed sunlight in the form of chemical energy (food) in a fossil-free world will require a sufficiency of people spread across our broad landscape . . . If (this) is right, rural communities throughout the world would need to fill up again just to feed the 6.5 billion people alive today, much less the 10 billion or so that are expected by the year 2050. . . . It has been estimated that to eliminate the need for (fuel) imports from the Middle East it would be necessary to produce 50 billion gallons of ethanol annually—which would require that half the country's usable farmland would need to be devoted to corn, resulting in significant and politically unpopular increases in food prices.

"Environmentalists complain that ethanol consumes about as much energy to make as it produces and that ethanol plants deplete aquifers, cause air pollution, and pollute water supplies," writes former First Lady Rosalynn Carter. "Sustainable agriculture presents an opportunity to rethink the importance of family farms and rural communities. Economic development policies are needed that encourage more diversified agricultural production on family farms as a foundation for healthy economies in rural communities."

Although rural poverty remains a problem, the situation has been improving, at least a tad. Rural counties still have poverty rates almost 25% higher than urban counties and account for almost 90% of all of the "persistent poverty" counties, defined by the US Department of Agriculture as counties that have experienced poverty rates above 20% for the past 30 years.

The term "economic gardening" refers to planting many seeds in order to grow the local economy in the hope that some will bear fruit. Small towns can romance the rising creative class or the "achievers" to settle in rural areas by developing more local amenities, with loan-forgiveness programs or land at reduced prices. We need to awaken America to the serious challenges facing rural America and create a national movement to sustainable agriculture and green energy in order to prepare our rural areas to compete globally. Rural America should be at the center of the drive for energy independence; it just makes sense. Solar energy fields, wind farms, and grains for alternative fuels all provide ample opportunity for innovation and economic growth in our rural areas. The politics of industrial farming has caused farming monocultures of grains and meat. Putting all our eggs in few agricultural baskets ignores the concept of crop diversity, which helps with soil nutrients and increases dependence on fossil fuels. The consequences for individual health and the environment are disastrous.

Maintaining a productive workforce means paying workers a living wage rather than a low minimum wage, and combating underemployment (the lack of employing people according to their education and ability), and providing them with sufficient hours or work in order to make a living on which they can be self-sufficient.

In conclusion, goals for economic development in rural areas should encourage small business development, entrepreneurship, niche industry and markets, cooperative regional efforts, and tourism, including ecotourism, agritourism, voluntourism, and cultural tourism. In order to use agriculture as economic development, rural America needs to find solutions to infrastructure obstacles such as transportation and affordable housing/lodging. Whatever direction our federal, state, and local governments take, the key to any successes will be what happens at the small-town level. True change starts on the grassroots level.

References

Addressing Mental Health Workforce Needs in Underserved Rural Areas: Accomplishments and Agriculture is Vital to New York's Economy. (2015). Overland Park, KS: National Crop Insurance Services.

Affordable Care Act Provisions Affecting the Rural Elderly (ACAPARE). (December, 2011). *National Advisory Committee on Rural Health and Human Services*.
Alliance for Health Reform (AHR). *Essentials of Health Policy: A Sourcebook for Journalists and Policymakers*. www.sourcebook.allhealth.org.
Bagalman, E. (2016). *The Helping Families in Mental Health Crisis Reform Act of 2016*. Washington, DC: Congressional Research Service.
Bailey, C., Jensen, L., & Ransom, E. (2014). *Rural America in a Globalizing World*. Morgantown: West Virginia University Press.
Barlett, P. F. (1993). *American Dreams, Rural Realities: Family Farms in Crisis*. Chapel Hill: University of North Carolina Press.
Brown, D. L., & Schafft, K. (2011). *Rural People and Communities*. Malden, MA: Polity Press.
Brown, D., & Swanson, L. (Eds.). (2003). *Challenges for Rural America in the Twenty-First Century*. University Park: Pennsylvania State University Press.
Carr, P. J., & Kefalas, M. J. (2009). *Hollowing Out the Middle: The Rural Brain Drain and What It Means for America*. Boston: Beacon Press.
Carter, R. (2010). *Within Our Reach: Ending the Mental Health Crisis*. Emmaus, PA: Rodale Books.
Castle, E. (Ed.). (1995). *The Changing American Countryside: Rural People and Places*. Lawrence: University Press of Kansas.
Cloke, P., Marsden, T., & Mooney, P. H. (Eds.). (2006). *Handbook of Rural Studies*. Thousand Oaks, CA: Sage.
Cornell University. (2010). *Poverty, Local and Regional Government, Energy, Economic and Workforce Development, Agriculture and Food Systems*. Ithaca, NY. www.cornell.edu.
Danbom, D. H. (2006). *Born in the Country: A History of Rural America*. Baltimore: Johns Hopkins University Press.
Davidson, O. G. (1996). *Broken Heartland: The Rise of America's Rural Ghetto*. Iowa City: University of Iowa Press.
Duncan, C. (1999). *Worlds Apart: Why Poverty Persists in Rural America*. New Haven, CT: Yale University Press.
Elder, G., & Conger, R. (Eds.). (2000). *Children of the Land: Adversity and Success in Rural America*. Chicago: University of Chicago Press.
Fitchen, J. (1991). *Endangered Spaces, Enduring Places*. Boulder, CO: Westview Press.
Flora, C. B., & Flora, J. L. (2008). *Rural Communities, Legacy and Change* (3rd ed.). Philadelphia, PA: Watershed Media.
A Short History and Summary of the Farm Bill. (2016) Arlington, VA: Farm Policy Facts. www.farmpolicyfacts.org.
Thomas, A., Lowe, B., Fulkerson, G., & Smith, P. (2011). *Critical Rural Theory: Structure, Space, Culture*. New York: Lexington Books.
University of California—Davis, Small Farm Program. (Fall, 1999). *Agricultural Policies and the Future of U.S. Family Farming*. Division of Agriculture and Natural Resources, University of California, Davis.
Wood, R. E. (2008). *Survival of Rural America: Small Victories and Bitter Harvests*. Lawrence: University Press of Kansas.

17 Technological Innovations in Rural Mental Health Services

Many are the technological innovations that have begun to improve access, availability, affordability, and acceptability of mental health services while reducing stigma. Telepsychology is the main innovation, but as any solution does, it comes with its own issues and challenges. License portability and confidentiality issues are just a few of these challenges.

Telepsychology

Although many rural residents do not have access to high-speed internet services, one of the fastest growing solutions to the rural mental health dilemma is the use of technology to bridge the geographic gap by allowing visits and assessments to happen virtually. Sometimes referred to as tele-behavioral health, it has a wide range of applications and some drawbacks. It started as an obvious outgrowth of the telehealth movement rather than an evidence-based treatment, however it is gaining ground in the latter venue.

And the great news is that as of January 1, 2015, Medicare added psychotherapy services to the list of telehealth services for residents who live in rural Health Professional Shortage Areas (HPSAs). The reimbursement rate is equivalent to an office visit.

From the professional's standpoint, it can allow the expansion of normal office hours, easy consultations with other specialists, and greater availability to share their specialty. One of the most obvious uses for teleconferencing is for educational purposes. Rural practitioners could participate more regularly in conferences, webinars, continuing education, and college coursework without having to travel long distances. The assumption is that the standard of care professionals provide would be the same as if the meeting were in person. However, like any other technological application, it creates issues of confidentiality according to standards under the Health Insurance Portability and Accountability Act of 1996 (HIPAA).

Some additional benefits for professionals include a decreased feeling of professional isolation and a greater likelihood of patients showing up (because in some cases they can access services from their home). It is easier to monitor patients for issues that may not warrant an appointment. This methodology also makes it easier to provide services from local community sites such as schools, offices, and residential treatment for patient continuity. They can also possibly increase the retention rate of remote employees and reduce time away from other clinical responsibilities. Interestingly enough, other technological methods have reportedly been used in mental health care, such as instant messaging, video conferencing, and audio conferencing. It is critical, as with in-person treatment, that the provider states clear expectations of service and provides the same level of care as they would in person. As stated previously, the inconsistency of reimbursement policies makes implementing these interventions more complicated. And to further complicate things, no two states are alike in their definition of or regulation of telehealth in general (for physical or emotional issues). It is my contention that students of mental health need to be versed in telehealth issues, possibilities, and regulations so they can help the profession increase access to mental health care in rural areas.

Two of the largest applications for telepsychology include hospitals and schools. Much more advocacy is needed for use in schools, as this methodology could be a much needed service to supplement overloaded mental health workers in schools across the country. Take the examples of crisis intervention, natural disasters, and specialized grief counseling—all of these could be easily provided via telepsychology methods with the staff doing the groundwork before and after the tele-intervention. In addition, because prescribers are rare in rural areas, it could provide a cost-effective way to assess for medication needs and maintenance.

In hospital emergency departments, where as many as 80% of patients with behavioral health conditions seek help, the emergency room staff is trained in some basic mental health crisis interventions, but their primary function is to address physical needs. According to the Alliance for Health Reform (AHR), as many as 70% of these patients are discharged without care. It is my experience that few rural hospitals have a mental health professional on staff for more than outpatient planning. Having a professional available to work with a patient's family during an emergency, and working with patients during their stay, should not be a luxury; it should be an important part of treating the whole person. Whether urban or rural, a patient's mental health and that of their loved ones should be offered as part of a regular treatment plan.

The AHR also reports that untreated mental illness is not only a major factor in homelessness and incarceration, but also has a significant impact on costs and overall health outcomes. Patients with these diagnoses tend to use more medical resources, are more likely to be hospitalized for medical conditions, and are readmitted to the hospital more frequently. Several members of Congress are calling for a major overhaul to the nation's mental health system. There are several areas of agreement in a wide variety of proposals, including expanding access to care, clarifying how HIPAA applies to mental health services, promoting electronic health record use, boosting the number of providers in underserved areas, and creating new federal leadership for behavioral health care.

Challenges in Telepsychology

According to Stamm, research shows that there are four major challenges that appear repeatedly when telehealth is discussed. They include evidence of its effectiveness, reimbursement, license and regulatory issues, and digital issues. Telehealth relies on high-speed internet connections, which many rural areas do not have. Telehealth also brings up licensing issues. Should the practitioner be licensed in their own state of origin or in the state the client is in? This is a slippery slope, because each state has its own firm credentialing policies and requirements. Not to mention, there are potential risks of confidentiality breaches through hacking.

HIPAA concerns regarding confidentiality over the internet are an ongoing issue, and are changing all the time. Therefore, practitioners need to rely on basic ethical concepts. For example, recording a therapy session, which could occur for a variety of reasons, could create legal and interpersonal complications. Would the recording fall under the category of session notes, which are given special protection under HIPAA? There is little guidance available for practitioners performing emergency tele-mental health services, and also for disaster mental health services. As the technology continues to develop and its use spreads, standards need to be developed addressing administrative regulation, passwords, encryption, and other security measures, transmitting, and technical standards.

License portability is one of the important issues in the development of telehealth use. But license portability goes beyond improving the efficiency and effectiveness of electronic mental health services. Overcoming unnecessary licensing barriers to cross-state practice has a dual function. It is seen by some as part of a general solution to workforce shortages and improve access to health care services. It is also seen as a way of improving the efficiency of the licensing system in this country so that scarce resources can be better used in the disciplinary and enforcement activities of state boards, rather than in duplicative licensing processes. The primary purpose of licensing health care professionals is to protect the public from incompetent or unethical practitioners. Over the years, the basic standards for various types of medical professional licenses have become fairly uniform across the states. The responsibility for overseeing licensure of all kinds has historically been given to each state. Some health policy experts have been calling for the federal government to enact national licensing standards for a long list of mental health professions that would set the bar, equalize the playing field, and hopefully alleviate the shortage of mental health professionals in rural areas.

Technophobia, as I call it, causes some barriers to this form of treatment. It stands to reason that the younger generations are more tech-friendly and savvy than older generations because many of them have used computers most of their lives. It has also been theorized that men, who have a high rate of turning away from mental health services, might find the use of technology more appealing, especially because it is one step removed in a sense. In addition to the phobia, there is a strong perception that implementation of these technological methods will be difficult because of the technology itself and possible accidental confidentiality breaches. Another barrier to telepsychology includes reimbursement issues. Currently, each state is responsible for creating and implementing their own "tele" policies. As with anything else, this presents regulatory challenges. At present, these are very inconsistent within and between states, and they bring up a tangle of licensing portability issues. Few states have licensing reciprocity in the mental health realm, creating the question: can a provider from one state treat a tele-patient from another state that has different licensing regulations? And, that brings up a larger question: would it benefit the mental health system to have federal licensing regulations rather than each state having its own? I venture to say that it would.

Telemedicine can be used for much more than therapy. It can be used for case management, medication management, psychiatric consultations, psychiatric referrals, professional development, and the supervision mental health professionals are required to engage in regularly. It can act as a lifeline by providing immediate support to those in the heat of a crisis and remain a support in the aftermath.

Outreach to educate communities should be expanded to include offering weekly therapy opportunities in local nursing homes, using local fairs and festivals to have a table with educational materials and someone to explain, answer questions, and talk about available community services and resources. Staff could also provide valuable community outreach by offering presentations to other kinds of professionals and organizations within the community, such as church groups, library programs, civic groups, and parents' groups. The list of topics that could be helpful to community members is as broad as their imaginations. Suggestions include domestic violence, trauma and post-traumatic responses, depression, suicide, drug and alcohol abuse, attachment disorders, aging, attention deficit hyperactivity disorder (ADHD), and parenting skills.

Although the federal government continues to issue grants to rural communities to make high-speed internet access available to all its citizens, rural areas continue to lag far behind in its availability. The Obama administration's American Recovery and Reinvestment Act of 2009 (ARRA) provides, among many other things, money to encourage the use of electronic medical records. Here again, rural areas lag behind urban areas in the receipt and use of these tools.

Many rural citizens rely on their local libraries for internet access and many of those libraries are only open part time. Therefore, the growth in telepsychology has to happen, for the present moment, within medical facilities where such access is available. And it remains to be seen what the cost-effectiveness of telepsychology actually is.

References

Bird, D. C., Dempsey, P., & Hartley, D. (2001). *Efforts to Address Mental Health Workforce Needs in Underserved Rural Areas.* University of Southern Maine, Institute for Health Policy, Maine Rural Health Research Center (Working Paper #23).

Centers for Disease Control and Prevention. (2011). *Public Health Action Plan to Integrate Mental Health Promotion and Mental Illness Prevention With Chronic Disease Prevention. 2011–2015.* Atlanta, GA: US Department of Health and Human Services.

Coalition for Mental Health Reform. (July 6, 2016). *Concerns With the Helping Families in Mental Health Crisis Act of 2015—passed in the House of Representatives.*

Cornell University. (2010). *Poverty, Local and Regional Government, Energy, Economic and Workforce Development, Agriculture and Food Systems.* Ithaca, NY. www.cornell.edu.

Hartley. D., Bird, D., Lambert, D., & Coffin, J. (November, 2002). *The Role of Community Mental Health Centers as Rural Safety Net Providers.* Portland: University of Southern Maine, Edmund S. Muskie School of Public Service, Maine Rural Health Research Center (Working Paper #30).

Hartley, D., Ziller, E., Lambert, D., Loux, S., & Bird, D. (October, 2002). *State Licensure Laws and the Mental Health Professions: Implications for the Rural Mental Health Workforce.* Portland: University of Southern Maine, Edmund S. Muskie School of Public Service, Maine Rural Health Research Center (Working Paper #29).

Jameson, J. P., & Blank, M. B. (2007). The role of clinical psychology in rural mental health services. Defining problems and developing solutions. *Clinical Psychology: Science and Practice,* 14, 283–298.

Kennedy Forum. (2016). *Navigating the New Frontier of Mental Health and Addiction: A Guide for the 115th Congress.* www.parityregistry.org; www.thekennedyforum.org; www.paritytrack.org.

Kennedy, P. J. (2015). *A Common Struggle: A Personal Journey Through the Past and Future of Mental Illness and Addiction.* New York: Blue Rider Press.

Layard, R., & Clark, D. M. (2015). *Thrive: How Better Mental Health Care Transforms Lives and Saves Money.* Princeton, NJ: Princeton University Press.

Manderscheid, R. (March 23, 2015). *Stigma Kills: On the Five "P's" of Inclusion and Social Justice.* www.nacbhdd.org.

Manderscheid, R. (June 7, 2016). Helping rural counties keep abreast of urban counterparts. *Behavioral Healthcare Magazine.* www.behavioral.net.

Neufeld, J., Case, R., & Serricchio, M. (2012). *Walk-in Telemedicine Clinics Improve Access and Efficiency: A Program Evaluation From the Perspective of a Rural Community Mental Health Center.* Washington, DC, *Rural Mental Health,* Fall/Winter.

New Freedom Commission on Mental Health. (2003). *Achieving the Promise: Transforming Mental Health Care in America.* Final. DHHS Pub. Co. SMA-03-3832. Rockville, MD.

Obama, B. (September 6, 2011). *Establishment of the White House Rural Council, Executive Order #13575.* Washington, DC: Office of the Federal Register. www.hsdl.org.

Ranier, J. P. (2010). The road much less travelled: Treating rural and isolated clients. *Journal of Clinical Psychology: In Session*, 66(5), 475–478.
Rural Policy Research Institute. (2016). www.rupri.org.
Sawyer, D., Gale, J., & Lambert, D. (2006). Rural *and Frontier Mental and Behavioral Health Care: Barriers, Effective Policy Strategies, and Best Practices.* Washington, DC: National Association for Rural Mental Health.
Schank, J., & Skovholt, T. (2006). *Ethical Practice in Small Communities: Challenges and Rewards for Psychologists.* Washington, DC: American Psychological Association.
Smith, A. (2003). Rural mental health counseling: One example of practicing what the research preaches. *Journal of Rural Community Psychology*, E6(2), Fall.
Stamm, B. H. (Ed.). (2003*). Rural Behavioral Health Care.* Washington, DC: American Psychological Association.
Townsend, W. (2010). Recovery services in rural settings, strengths and challenges influencing behavioral healthcare service delivery. *Rural Mental Health*, 34(1),23–32.
Vandiver, V. L. (2013). *Best Practices in Community Mental Health.* Chicago: Lyceum Books.
Weigel, D. (2009). *The Challenges of Rural Clinical Mental Health Counseling.* Weitz, Germany: VDM Verlag.
Ziller, E. (2002). *State Licensure Laws and the Mental Health Professions: Implications for the Rural Mental Health Workforce.* Cutler Institute for Health and Social Policy, Portland, ME.

18 Looking Forward
Collaborative Possibilities

About 85% of counties in the United States have either no mental health services at all, or they are inadequate. The mental health needs of rural Americans are huge, and while there are some promising new approaches to improving our mental healthcare system being implemented, there is still a long distance to travel in creating an adequate, quality, affordable system for all. Some involve creating new positions, and others involve constructing new paradigms. Decarceration is one new paradigm, but there are many others. In 2008, The President's New Freedom Commission on Mental Health's Rural Subcommittee outlined potential areas for improvement, most of which have yet to be put into place. There are also other new programs and ideas on the horizon. Some require collaboration between people, agencies, and the creation of more multidisciplinary teams. Many require grants, and grant writing and grant resources are discussed briefly at the end of this chapter.

According to the National Rural Health Association, the mental health needs of rural Americans are immense and the implementation of adequate services in rural areas is a critical national health imperative. Three of the most promising approaches to improving our mental health care system are integrated care services, telehealth technologies, and school and home-based interventions. Over 40% of individuals with mental health needs start to seek treatment in a primary care setting. School is also a natural place for mental health interventions given that nearly all children in rural areas attend school and transportation to schools is already in place. Many counties are creating a position called a family support specialist, which involves a therapist going into the home and working with the entire family on their own turf. These are master's level professionals who are either counselors or social workers. This is proving to be an effective treatment methodology. Much can be gained from seeing a family interact in its own surroundings. It also eliminates transportation issues that are often obstacles to treatment in rural areas, and reduces the possibility of stigma for seeking care by not being seen at the local clinic.

Some states, such as New Hampshire, require licensees from each profession to obtain 25 hours of collaboration with other types of mental health professionals for each renewal year. Some examples of collaborations include small group meetings, consultation, study groups, and telephone conferences. Collaboration is the way of the future as funds dwindle and need grows.

Another concept worth exploring is that of making the mental health advocate a professional role rather than a volunteer role, with a credentialing process. These advocates would do as they are now—providing a level of support to those who need a lower support level. Sometimes called peer specialists, these advocates provide a grassroots level of reaching out to people in need and bypassing stigma. In addition, they could help those in need protect their rights, and empower them to make their own decisions regarding their care, help them access needed services, and help educate the public at large. They could help ease the transition from prison or jail, as well as help with unburdening the overcrowded jail while providing specific support in the hopes of lowering recidivism. In the growing movement for decarceration, these advocates can help make the difference in recidivism by guiding people through the ever complex network we call the mental health system. A new type of professional mental health advocate is needed to ensure that appropriate public policies are created that protect the rights of consumers as well as giving them accurate information on their options. Advocacy is the current bridge for traveling from distress to diagnosis to treatment and follow-up, as well as routes to prevention through public education. Some envision that the mental health advocate could be a bachelor's level professional, or a graduate of a 1-year certificate program. These advocates could perform much needed services in mental health clinics, nursing homes, hospice settings, schools, judicial settings, psychiatric hospitals, and anywhere a mental health professional would seek employment. They could also be trained to give public presentations to educate the public about mental health issues while reducing stigma. It would be highly cost-effective to add this type of position into the mental health mix. The federal government needs to appropriate additional funding for more mental health research, perhaps in the form of grants to colleges, universities, and other research facilities and organizations.

About 85% of counties in the United States have either no mental health services at all, or they are inadequate. Federal and state agencies must make a deliberate effort to balance grant and contract awards between urban and rural counties, and they must develop specific programs for rural counties that are "rural-centric." Rural areas may benefit from technical assistance in order to take advantage of these grant opportunities. Perhaps requiring grant and contract announcements that are specifically directed toward rural counties would make a significant improvement. Federal and state lawmakers must work closely together to train and provide motivation for behavioral health providers to live and work in rural areas. Workforce shortages are now at crisis levels. They also need to work together to implement telehealth outreach for rural counties. In many cases, this means installing technological infrastructure in the form of cell phone towers and fiber-optic cable.

Most rural communities don't have a community center or recreation center. Because schools are the centerpiece of most rural communities, let's use our schools for more community recreation and family events. Organizations such as Mental Health America (MHA) have a website (www.mhascreening.org) with online screenings people can take to help provide a context for symptoms and help determine the need for help to people who are hesitant to seek mental health treatment. This resource currently hosts screenings for depression, anxiety, bipolar disorder, post-traumatic stress disorder (PTSD), and alcohol and substance use, as well as a youth and parent screen and a work health survey. More of these kinds of screenings made readily available could help countless people to the tipping point of seeking help.

In states that have land grant universities, or other universities that are willing to participate, information networks can be funneled through these institutions for easy dissemination to professionals and to the public. These institutions and many others are actually doing research that is critical to helping improve the rural mental health system and have their fingers on the results for broadcasting. More networks like this need to be formed, funded, and publicized. These institutions can help provide training in grant writing, training on rural issues for professionals, needs assessments, technical assistance, and public education seminars.

In 2004, the President's New Freedom Commission on Mental Health's Rural Subcommittee listed potential areas in which improvements can be made in rural mental health. Most of them have not been put into place or still need significant improvement. They include:

- Short response ties for grant funding applications and requests for grant proposals that put rural programs and human resource shortages at a disadvantage in assembling the resources required to prepare a competitive submission.
- Matching fund requirements that do not take into account the available resource pool in rural markets (e.g., programs on Native American reservations that are required to show the same non-federal match as all programs, when most health resources available are federally funded).
- Lack of research and demonstration of rural-specific evidence-based practices.
- Continued focus on specialty-driven practice and policy, when the rural literature supports a generalist model.
- The assumption that metropolitan-tested policies and practices only need to be "downsized" to fit rural area needs. For example, when it comes to meeting a client's needs, the urban assumption is that the obligation is to meet the client's need for specialized mental health services and refer them to other supportive services to meet other needs. The rural reality is that the obligation is to meet the full range of mental health and supportive needs of clients because no other supportive services are available.

Many are the needs for research in rural and frontier areas. For example, there is a high need for researching job satisfaction and ways to provide mental health services to in areas that need access. Tele-mental health is another area still in its infancy that would benefit greatly from research assessing its effectiveness and whether or not it can offer other applications successfully. Assessments themselves that are used to measure efficacy of treatment need to be studied to confirm validity and reliability as instruments.

Mental Health First Aid is a program that is gaining popularity. The Mental Health First Aid Act of 2013 authorized funding to educate parents, first responders, faith leaders, and the general population to understand and respond to signs of mental illness and substance use disorders, including risk factors and warning signs. It also teaches people how to de-escalate crisis situations safely and initiate referrals to mental health and substance abuse resources. The program uses a 5-step action plan to reach out to those in crisis and connect them to professionals and peers. To become certified, people take an 8- to 12-hour class. Funded through federal grants, there is also a special youth version of the program aimed to teach concerned citizens how to help teens and young adults. The mental health program's rural efforts address the unique characteristics of rural areas. First Aid is a collaborative effort involving over two dozen agencies. More about Mental Health First Aid can be found at www.thenationalcouncil.org.

Every medical examination should include a brain health evaluation, starting with the depression screen, which, although it is now fully covered under the Affordable Care Act, many doctors still aren't using it. Mental health screenings need to be tied to an aggressive plan of early diagnosis and intervention.

For professionals, part of their continuing education activities should include courses on new developments in brain health, and this should be expanded for attorneys, judges, and law enforcement and medical professionals. Research is teaching us more about the elaborate workings of the brain all the time.

According to Wood, Hillary Rodham Clinton proposed federal support for a wide range of rural initiatives, including expanding rural internet access, promoting ethanol and other crop-based alternative fuels, funding efforts to attract doctors to rural areas, rebuilding downtowns, and creating tourist attractions. Noting that most rural Americans aren't farmers or ranchers, she also endorsed more federal support for rural economic development, not just agriculture.

According to former Congressman Patrick Kennedy, the only way we can have modern facilities for integrated medical mental health and care for people with addiction is if the federal government reforms the old Institutions for Mental Disease (IMD) exclusion to the Medicaid law in the Social Security Act once and for all. He explains that in the 1960s, the IMD exclusion was meant to prevent dilapidated institutions from refilling their beds after Medicaid/Medicare was passed. But in past decades it has been the single largest handicap to quality mental health care. The exclusion limits old and new facilities with more than 16 inpatient mental health beds and more than 51% of patients with mental illness from getting reimbursement from Medicaid for patients between the ages of 22 and 64—which, by the way, is the largest portion of our population. This dramatically limits the number of inpatient beds for mental health available to patients in America, and has a horrible downward spiraling effect through all of mental health care.

Congress should increase funding for National Health Service Corps scholarship and loan repayments in order to increase the supply of behavioral and mental health professionals. They could also provide tax credits for these practitioners, which would still give them an economic boost and contribute significantly to job retention rates in underserved rural areas. The Centers for Medicare and Medicaid Services should remove payment obstacles to and improve reimbursement for evidence-based approaches to integrating specialty behavioral care in primary care, including care management services, the use of standardized outcome measures, and the regular caseload review and consultation by a designated psychiatric consultant done by phone or video.

States should require interdisciplinary training in evidence-based integrated care for mental health specialists and primary care providers as part of continuing medical education for state medical licensure. Rural issues must be brought to the attention of the workforce as a whole, as early in their training as possible.

Congress should amend the Health Information Technology for Economic and Clinical Health (HITECH) Act and extend financial incentives for the meaningful use of electronic health records to mental health and addiction treatment providers and facilities. In order to comply with HIPAA (Health Insurance Portability and Accountability Act of 1996) regulations in the high-tech world, standards need to be made clear in order to protect patient confidentiality in the ever changing world of computer hacking and the like.

The Presidential Commission on Mental Health identified rural areas as underserved and a priority for future research and service programs. It seems important to make certain that what is positive and unique about rural areas is preserved and that rural issues are addressed in ways that are appropriate to honoring both the land and the population.

Senator Lamar Alexander, the chair of the US Senate Committee on Health, Education, Labor and Pensions, announced in February 2016 that one of his goals for 2016 was to develop and pass a long-awaited mental health reform bill. Simultaneously, Congressman Gene Greene of Texas, the ranking member of the Health Subcommittee of the US House Energy and Commerce Committee, and five of his colleagues introduced the Comprehensive Behavioral Health Reform and Recovery Act of 2016. The bill, which at the time of this writing is stalled in Congress, is a bipartisan effort that will provide an essential framework for the Senate to use to introduce similar legislation. According to Ron Manderscheid at the National Association for Rural Mental Health, this bill can address the fundamental needs for mental health and substance use infrastructure and services at the county, state, and federal levels. Importantly, this bill also recognizes the critical role played by trauma, recovery, and peers in behavioral health care, and the importance of the appropriate infrastructure within the workforce.

According to the bill's main author Congressman Gene Green, any efforts at mental health care reform must transform the system from the ground up, and this legislation provides such a foundation to start from as mental health reform discussions continue in Congress. This bill includes key provisions to update the use of Medicaid for care while removing barriers to home- and community-based mental health services.

In addition, a new bill called the Accountable Health Communities (AHC) model addresses a critical gap between clinical care and community services in the current delivery system by testing whether systematically identifying and addressing the health-related social needs of people impacts total health care costs, improves health, and quality care. A recent landmark event signaling the transition to include social services in the partnership of physical and mental health model is the new grant announcement that extends Medicaid financial participation to aid in the integration of services. This is a landmark step never before taken in the 51-year history of Medicaid.

Because the Wellstone-Domenici Mental Health Parity Act will only help those who work for a company with more than 50 employees, and this is a minority of rural residents, we need to continue to advocate strongly for the millions of farmers, ranchers, and other self-employed people and those employed in small rural businesses. This is what was originally promised in the President's New Freedom Commission Rural Subcommittee: rural parity, meaning that rural residents be provided the same access to mental health range of services that urban folks receive.

Creating an Assistant Secretary for Mental Health within the federal government is another idea deserving of serious consideration. A similar idea with merit is to establish a White House Office of Mental Health Policy and Program Coordination, similar to the Office of National Drug Control Policy, which has operated within the executive office successfully for years.

According to Rural Behavioral Health Programs with Promising Practices, many rural providers have identified and implemented novel and potentially effective solutions to the accessibility, availability, and acceptability barriers to rural behavioral health care, but there is very little documentation and exchange of information as to what has worked or failed to work across rural areas. Services such as the Substance Abuse and Mental Health Services Administration's (SAMHSA's) National Registry of Evidence-Based Programs (EBP) and Practices (NREPP) exist to share information about EBPs, but these services are limited EBPs that are not tailored to or tested in rural populations and may not generalize well to rural communities. Rural behavioral health programs with extensive community support tend to succeed and grow because whole communities are invested in improving behavioral health. I would add that the dissemination of information needs to be improved greatly. The seeds of many great ideas are out there in rural communities with no way to share and have other communities help test their viability. Perhaps smaller regional conferences held at regular intervals would help with the dissemination process while also offering continuing education/professional development, which to many is a perk. This would be a cost-effective way to accomplish many goals at once.

President Obama started 2016 by pressuring Republicans in Congress to make good on their promise to fix the broken mental health system, which they have frequently blamed for gun violence. He called for a half billion dollars in new mental health spending, reminding Congress of their failed promise to pass a mental health reform bill since they pledged to do so back in 2013 after the Newtown, Connecticut, mass shooting.

In March 2016, SAMHSA announced a new grant challenge to help aid in the development of a mobile application that provides additional recovery support to patients receiving treatment for opioid abuse. Legislators need to know that national policies are often based on urban models (think: urbancentric), and are not always appropriate in rural areas.

We must mandate that all schools have licensed counselors so that emotional literacy and self-knowledge begins at an early age so that it is seen as equal to physical health issues and provides students with tools in their "emotional toolboxes" that they can carry with them for life. It's no secret that the No Child Left Behind Act had us focusing more time and attention on student achievement at the expense of other kinds of learning, such as social/emotional support. A student who is surrounded by an emotional fog is not able to learn. His brain chemistry is wrapped up in survival, in trying to regain equilibrium, and in self-protection. Students in these circumstances—and they are a population that grows exponentially every year—are caught up in Maslow's hierarchy of needs, seeking the most basic of needs such as physiological, safety, love, and belonging before they can learn effectively. According to the National Association for Rural Mental Health (NARMH), in 2009, 21% of students are seen as experiencing signs and symptoms of a DSM-5 disorder during the course of a year. Only 20% of those with extreme impairments report receiving mental health services. Each youth whose emotional issues remain unresolved is at an increased risk of isolation, suicide, substance abuse, and violent acting out. In tough economic times, it is difficult to sell the concept of prevention. How can we help each and every child reach his/her full potential under these circumstances?

During the 2016 presidential election campaign, Hillary Clinton stated that mental health would be a top priority in her administration. She also stated that she would create a White House Conference on Mental Health during her first year in office. Donald Trump never mentioned mental health. According to Ron Manderscheid in *Behavioral Healthcare*, excellent evidence exists that Clinton addressed the appropriate topics. Her proposals included addressing the key topics of insurance parity, prevention and promotion, and care integration. Her proposals also demonstrated that she understands the current dilemmas confronting mental health. She identified large-scale incarceration of persons with mental illness, the dramatic rise in suicides, and the mental health workforce crisis as three additional topics for which urgent action is needed.

Much more attention must be paid to policies and programs at the state and local levels. The federal government must maintain a leading role in assuring that policy, programs, and funding innovations advance these rural opportunities. Educating the public is a key component of ensuring this growing collaboration for the benefit of us all.

Changing America's mental health system from its medical-oriented institutional thinking to a more modern, applicable model, one based on the principles of building on strengths toward recovery, will require a concerted effort from consumers and professionals working together to bring about changes in beliefs and practices at every level of the system—and at the same time, working to educate the public toward eliminating stigma. *It can be done.*

We should be looking to create an approach to mental health that consists of a multidisciplinary team including medical and nursing staff, psychologists, social workers, spiritual supports, and complementary treatments like healing touch, massage therapy, and neurofeedback that are evidence based. It should also include all the creative arts therapies, which are not yet covered by Medicaid, although they would be cost-effective in helping to prevent hospitalizations and improve the quality of life for patients. Art, music, drama, and movement therapies are also evidence based, and present alternative strategies to traditional talk therapy. The addition of nutritional counselors, healing touch, and massage therapy would also prove cost-effective if integrated into the team approach, and would help guide family members and loved ones through the quagmire of systems involved in a client's care while providing support, information, and other kinds of assistance. Providing a comprehensive education and support system would help them in dealing with their loved one's mental illness, available treatment options, and learning positive ways to communicate and react with a loved one who has a mental or physical illness. Support groups where families can interact with each other and learn from others in similar situations with their loved ones should be frequent and well publicized. Having useful printed information and resource materials on hand in emergency rooms for psychiatric emergencies is necessary. When families are in crisis, they should be able to get this level of support at once so that they can find ways to cope and be useful to the treatment team.

We should also be working toward the ability of various kinds of treatment providers to communicate via technological means in order to shorten the collaboration process. Colleges, universities, and national mental health organizations can offer more online classes or webinars, making it easier to keep current on trends and discoveries while eliminating the need for travel. Creating more respite havens for people experiencing stress, anxiety, and depression would help avoid the travel time and cost of crisis centers and psychiatric emergency rooms and hospitalizations. There they could receive support, encouragement, qualified services, and a safety plan. This would be the "least restrictive environment" for those with a mental health crisis. This would be a person-centered approach with coordination of a variety of services, including medical, psychiatric, psychosocial, and psychoeducational.

Another program we should aspire to is to have a Medicaid version of the waiver program for adults with mental illness that is similar to the Home and Community Based Service waiver that ends at age 21, the approximate age when many mental illnesses emerge. Also, traumatic brain injury services could be expanded in the same way.

Mental health clinics need to offer group as well as individual therapy, and many people can be enrolled in one or the other, and in some cases, both. While the one-on-one treatment model is important for personal attention, groups offer an opportunity for peers to learn from each other, providing validation and enhancing self-esteem and knowledge. Groups help raise awareness that one is not alone in having a mental illness, thereby reducing stigma and a sense of isolation.

The way of America's future economic growth, and to some extent the rest of the world, is dependent on an increasing interdependence and collaboration between rural and urban resources, cultures, and innovations. Therefore, it is essential that rurality be taken into greater consideration at the policy-making levels as well as the grassroots levels. And it is essential that there be an equal opportunity between urban and rural areas. The future of rural regions and the communities they are made up of will be largely determined by their innovation, entrepreneurship, and making the best use of their assets and resources. All policy considerations from the federal and state to the county and local community must include honoring our environment and stewardship of our planet. The quality of our land, air, water, and natural resources will determine our quality of life in the future.

Some other ideas for improving rural mental health services in rural America include the following. All require adequate funding, but would be cost-effective in the long term.

- Adding warm lines and crisis lines where they are lacking.
- Create centers that are "living room" models of recovery-based care. These are used as an attempt to de-medicalize centers as much as possible. They are for short-term use and include respite beds for overnight stays. Incoming patients are referred to as guests.
- Wellness recovery centers for individuals with longer term needs who can utilize such a center between hospital or jail discharge and their future arrangements. They claim a high success rate in diverting people from hospitalizations, making the model cost-effective and patient centered.
- Increase educational programs to teach first responders, clergy, and other community services mental health training for assessing and referring someone in a crisis.
- Develop, identify, and access funding to establish sustainable innovative recovery and wellness programs and community outreach. Using best practices, develop training and support to help with the retention of qualified staff and improve the 4 A's and S: access, acceptability, availability, affordability, and stigma.
- Partner with state and federal lawmakers to obtain funding and/or revisit funding streams for improving the rural mental health system by developing and implementing innovative programs.

- Have local stakeholders determine how available agencies can work more collaboratively.

In June 2017, a groundbreaking collaborative effort of four major professional counseling organizations aimed at improving access to quality mental health care nationwide resulted in a proposed uniform portability plan called the "National Counselor Licensure Endorsement Process." Their collective belief is that a uniform licensure endorsement process will:

- Significantly increase public access to qualified care.
- Establish minimum standards for safe practice.
- Reduce administrative burdens for state regulatory boards and licensees.
- Create consistency in licensure standards across state lines.
- Ensure protection of the public and the continued development of the profession.

To move the counseling profession toward unified educational standards, exam requirements and years required of post-graduate experience prior to licensure will address license reciprocity between states. We need more of this kind of collaboration in order to obtain more uniformity and license portability in order to meet the growing mental health needs of our nation.

A Word About Funding and Developing Promising Practices

In the Rural Behavioral Health Programs and Promising Practices Guide, there are several characteristics of successful programs that can be used to assess the strengths and weaknesses of a new or developing program. They include:

- Relevance/impact on rural behavioral health. Use mission statements to develop a mission for the program.
- Community engagement. The key is to realize others in the community are also interested in building connections.
- Ensuring the need will be met. Bringing a wide range of organizations and individuals together ensures meeting needs and contributes to sustainability.
- Getting stakeholders involved. Programs successful in engaging the community work hard to maintain these connections despite busy schedules, staff turnover, and lack of resources.
- Connecting with researchers and evaluators. These connections can be local or out-of-state. When applying for funding, include the cost of an outside evaluator.

- Capacity and documentation. Consider who the target population is, what are the main components of the program, location, times and dates, why the program is needed—the hole it fills in services. What are staff members' roles?
- Specifying details. It is important to document the program in as much detail as possible to ensure that someone else could replicate it based on the documentation alone.
- Marketing program services to communities. Can be done with a brochure, talks, giveaways (magnets, pens, etc.), presenting at conferences, and writing papers or articles in local publications.
- Sustainability and expansion. A word about funding. Grants are generally classified according to the entity that is offering the grant opportunity. Within each entity, there may be a number of different types of grants. The general classifications are federal, state, and private foundations.

At www.grants.gov, you can subscribe to email notifications to receive information about various types of grant opportunities, search using keywords, and read tips on effectively using the database and ways to seek technical assistance on completing federal grant forms. The Rural Assistance Center (www.racon line.org) is also a good source of grant and other information.

To identify state grants, check the state Health and Human Services website for in-subject areas. Opportunities vary between states. A good source for rural project funding is your state office of rural health (see listing at end of book).

To apply for a grant from a private foundation, there are online resources for searching grant opportunities; however, some require a fee. Once a grant opportunity has been identified, confirm you are eligible to apply for the program, identify necessary application requirements, and determine whether or not the purpose of the grant fits with the purpose and goals of the intended project. It is often helpful to talk with the grant project officer and then the community to engage support. Don't be afraid to ask them questions during the grant writing process.

The most important characteristic of effective applications is that they have followed all the instructions completely. Be sure every "I" is dotted and every "T" crossed. It is sometimes possible to look at applications that have been funded and some that were not funded by asking the funding organization to provide an example. Successful grant applications are well written. Grant writing classes are available either at local colleges or universities or online. They are well worth the time and effort.

According to Smalley, Warren, and Rainer in *Rural Mental Health*, viewing rurality as a cultural issue rather than geographic issue could lead to a dramatic shift in the way rural issues are viewed, and thus could help facilitate fruitful discussions with a consistent meaning. This, in turn, could have a vast and profound effect on delivering much needed, quality mental health services to the heartland of our country.

> **Quotes on the Nation's Heartland**
>
> The troubles in America's Heartland are symptoms of much larger problems in our society . . . with its roots deep in the land.
> —Osha Gray Davidson *(Broken Heartland)*
>
> Because we know that there is a huge gap between the discovery or development of a useful intervention and its adoption in community-based settings, the biggest mental health research problem we face today is not the advancement of knowledge, but translating that research into practice more quickly.
> —Rosalynn Carter

References

Bagalman, E. (2016). *The Helping Families in Mental Health Crisis Reform Act of 2016*. Washington, DC: Congressional Research Service.

Bailey, C., Jensen, L., & Ransom, E. (2014). *Rural America in a Globalizing World*. Morgantown: West Virginia University Press.

Bain, S. F. (November, 2010). Itinerant counseling services for rural communities: A win/win opportunity. *Journal of Rural Community Psychology*, E13(1).

Bird, D. C., Dempsey, P., & Hartley, D. (2001). *Efforts to Address Mental Health Workforce Needs in Underserved Rural Areas*. University of Southern Maine, Institute for Health Policy, Maine Rural Health Research Center (Working Paper #23).

Brown, D., & Swanson, L. (Eds.). (2003). *Challenges for Rural America in the Twenty-First Century*. University Park: Pennsylvania State University Press.

Butler, C., Butler, J., & Gasteyer, S. (2016). *Rural Communities: Legacy and Change* (5th ed.). Boulder, CO: Westview Press.

Butler, S. S., & Kaye, L. (2003). *Gerontological Social Work in Small Townsend and Rural Communities*. Binghamton, NY: Haworth Press.

Carr, P. J., & Kefalas, M. J. (2009). *Hollowing Out the Middle: The Rural Brain Drain and What It Means for America*. Boston: Beacon Press.

Carter, R. (2010). *Within Our Reach: Ending the Mental Health Crisis*. Emmaus, PA: Rodale Books.

Castle, E. (Ed.). (1995). *The Changing American Countryside: Rural People and Places*. Lawrence: University Press of Kansas.

Census.gov/geo/tiger/glossry2.html.

Centers for Disease Control and Prevention. (2011). *Public Health Action Plan to Integrate Mental Health Promotion and Mental Illness Prevention With Chronic Disease Prevention. 2011–2015*. Atlanta, GA: US Department of Health and Human Services.

Childs, A. W., & Melton, G. B. (1983). *Rural Psychology*. New York: Plenum Press.

Cloke, P., Marsden, T., & Mooney, P. H. (Eds.). (2006). *Handbook of Rural Studies*. Thousand Oaks, CA: Sage.

Coalition for Mental Health Reform. (July 6, 2016). *Concerns With the Helping Families in Mental Health Crisis Act of 2015—Passed in the House of Representatives.*

Cornell University. (2010). *Poverty, Local and Regional Government, Energy, Economic and Workforce Development, Agriculture and Food Systems.* Ithaca, NY. www.cornell.edu.

Davidson, O. G. (1996). *Broken Heartland: The Rise of America's Rural Ghetto.* Iowa City: University of Iowa Press.

Duncan, C. (1999). *Worlds Apart: Why Poverty Persists in Rural America.* New Haven, CT: Yale University Press.

Elder, G., & Conger, R. (Eds.). (2000). *Children of the Land: Adversity and Success in Rural America.* Chicago: University of Chicago Press.

Federal Office of Rural Health Policy (March 17, 2017). *Special Announcement—CDC on Rural Children and Mental Health.*

Flora, C.B., & Flora, J.L. (2008). *Rural Communities, Legacy and Change* (3rd ed.). Philadelphia, PA: Westview Press/Perseus Books.

Goldman, H.H., Buck, J.A., & Thompson, K. S. (2009). *Transforming Mental Health Services: Implementing the Federal Agenda for Change.* Arlington, VA: American Psychiatric Association.

Grantham, D. (February 1, 2017). National Association of County Behavioral Health and Developmental Disability Directors (NACBHDD). *The Challenge of Affordable Health Care: The ACA and Beyond.* Washington, DC.

Kennedy Forum. (2016). *Navigating the New Frontier of Mental Health and Addiction: A Guide for the 115th Congress.* www.parityregistry.org; www.thekennedyforum.org; www.paritytrack.org.

Kennedy Forum. (2017). *Issue Brief: Fixing Behavioral Health Care in America.* www.thekennedyforum.org.

Kennedy, P.J. (2015). *A Common Struggle: A Personal Journey Through the Past and Future of Mental Illness and Addiction.* New York: Blue Rider Press.

Manderscheid, R. (March 23, 2015). *Stigma Kills: On the Five "P's" of Inclusion and Social Justice.* www.nacbhdd.org.

Manderscheid, R. (June 7, 2016). Helping rural counties keep abreast of urban counterparts. *Behavioral Healthcare Magazine.* www.behavioral.net.

Manderscheid, R. (August 28, 2016). Last chance to pass mental health reform? *Behavioral Healthcare Magazine.* www.behavioral.net.

Manderscheid, R. (August 30, 2016). *Hillary Clinton Offers Excellent Mental Health Policy Proposals.* www.behavioral.net.

Manderscheid, R. (December 19, 2016). *Treatment and Housing for Persons With Serious Mental Illness.* www.naco.org.

Mental Health America. (August 29, 2016). *Statement by Paul Gionfriddo, President and CEO, Mental Health America.* mhapostmaster@mentalhealthamerica.net.

Mental Health and Rural America: 1994–2005. (2005). Washington, DC: Health Resources and Services Administration, Office of Rural Health Policy.

Mohatt, D. F. (2016). *Rural Mental Health: Challenges and Opportunities Caring for the Country.* Boulder, CO: Western Interstate Commission for Higher Education.

Morris, J. (2009, Summer). Marriage and family therapists expand access to mental health services in rural areas. *Journal of Rural Community Psychology*, E12(1).

Morris, J.A. (1997). *Practicing Psychology in Rural Settings.* Washington, DC: American Psychological Association.

New Freedom Commission on Mental Health. (2003). *Achieving the Promise: Transforming Mental Health Care in America*. Final. DHHS Pub. Co. SMA-03-3832. Rockville, MD.

Obama, B. (September 6, 2011). *Establishment of the White House Rural Council, Executive Order #13575*. Washington, DC: Office of the Federal Register. www.hsdl.org.

Office of the Assistant Secretary for Planning and Evaluation. Department of Health and Human Services. (January 11, 2017). *Continuing Progress on the Opioid Epidemic: The Role of the Affordable Care Act*. Rockville, MD.

Quinn, M. (September, 2016). *Rural America Finally Gets Mental Health Help*. www.governing.com/templates/gov_print_article.

Rural Policy Research Institute. (2016). www.rupri.org.

Sawyer, D., Gale, J., & Lambert, D. (2006). *Rural and Frontier Mental and Behavioral Health Care: Barriers, Effective Policy Strategies, and Best Practices*. Washington, DC: National Association for Rural Mental Health.

Schank, J., & Skovholt, T. (2006). *Ethical Practice in Small Communities: Challenges and Rewards for Psychologists*. Washington, DC: American Psychological Association.

Semuels, A. (June 2, 2016). The Greying of Rural America. *The Atlantic*.

Slama, K. (2004). Toward rural cultural competence. *Minnesota Psychologist*, 53(2), 6–13.

Smalley, K.B., Warren, J., & Rainer, J. (Eds.). (2012). *Rural Mental Health: Issues, Policies, and Best Practices*. New York: Springer.

Smalley, K.B., Yancey, C.T., Warren, J.C., Naufel, K., Ryan, R., & Pugh, J.L. (2010). Rural mental health and psychological treatment: A review for practitioners. *Journal of Clinical Psychology: In Session*, 66(5), 479–489.

Stamm, B.H. (Ed.). (2003). *Rural Behavioral Health Care*. Washington, DC: American Psychological Association.

US Department of Health and Human Services. (1999). Rockville, MD: Substance Abuse and Mental Health Services Administration. Promising Practices. Rockville, MD: Office of Rural Health Policy, Health Resources and Services Administration.

Van Hecke, S. (2012). *Behavioral Health Aides: A Promising Practice for Frontier Communities*. Silver City, NM: The National Center for Frontier Communities and Frontier and Rural Expert Panel.

Vandiver, V.L. (2103). *Best Practices in Community Mental Health*. Chicago: Lyceum Books.

Weigel, D. (2009). *The Challenges of Rural Clinical Mental Health Counseling*. Weitz, Germany: VDM Verlag.

Whitaker, R. (2010). *Anatomy of an Epidemic*. New York: Broadway Books.

Wilson, W., Bangs, A., & Hatting, T. (February, 2015). *The Future of Rural Behavioral Health*. National Rural Health Association Policy Brief. www.ruralhealthnet.org

Wiltz, T. (2016, October 20). Can the Arts Help Save Rural America? *The Huffington Post*.

Wood, R.E. (2008). *Survival of Rural America: Small Victories and Bitter Harvests*. Lawrence: University Press of Kansas.

Ziller, E. (2002). *State Licensure Laws and the Mental Health Professions: Implications For the Rural Mental Health Workforce*. Portland, ME: Cutler Institute for Health and Social Policy.

Mental Health Organizations

This list is far from exhaustive, but provides a good starting point for anyone wanting further information on rural mental health issues.

- Every state has its own office of alcohol and substance abuse as well as its own office of mental health. These can be found using any search engine.
- State and local government on the internet—guide to government-sponsored sites (www.piperinfo.com).
- American Fact Finder, the portal for the US Census Bureau (www.factfinder.census.gov).

Administration for Children and Families Office of Planning, Research and Evaluation

The Program Manager's Guide to Program Evaluation (www.acf.hhs.gov/programs).

American Association of Community Psychiatrists (AACP)

Helps community and public psychiatrists to develop and implement policies and high-quality practices that promote individual, family, and community resilience and recovery.

American Foundation for Suicide Prevention (AFSP)

Dedicated to funding research, developing prevention initiatives, and offering educational programs and conferences for survivors, mental health professionals, physicians, and the public.

CDC Evaluation Working Group

www.cdc.gov/eval/index

Center for Rural Affairs

145 Main Street
P.O. Box 136
Lyons, NE 68038
www.cfra.org

Center for Rural Mental Health Studies

University of Minnesota Medical School
420 Delaware Street, SE
Minneapolis, MN 55455
www.med.umn.edu/about/duluth-campus/center-rural-mental-health

Centers for American Indian and Alaska Native Health (CAIANH)

Colorado School of Public Health
13001 E. 17th Street
Mail Stop B11
Aurora, CO 80045
303-724-4585
Colorado.sph@ucdenver.edu

Centers for Disease Control and Prevention

1600 Clifton Avenue
Atlanta, GA 30329-4027
800-232-4636
www.cdc.gov

Centers for Medicare and Medicaid Services (CMS)

7500 Security Boulevard
Baltimore, MD 21244
877-267-2323
www.cms.gov

Consumer Organization and Networking Technical Assistance Center (CONTAC)

SAMHSA
5600 Fishers Lane
Rockville, MD 20857
877-726-4727

Drug Abuse Treatment Cost Analysis Program

www.datcap.com

Eastern Tennessee State University Department of Psychology

www.etsu.edu/cas/psychology/graduate/programs/clinicalphd/

Farm Policy Facts

P.O. Box 596
Arlington, VA 22216
www.farmpolicyfacts.org

FastStats—Center for Disease Control and Prevention

www.cdc.nchs.gov/nchs/fastats/default.htm

FedStats

www.fedstats.sites.usa.gov

Frontier Mental Health Services Resource Network

Western Interstate Commission for Higher Education, Mental Health
P.O. Box 9752
Boulder, CO 80301
303-541-0256
www.wiche.edu

Gay, Lesbian, and Straight Educational Network

www.glsen.org

Georgetown University Center for Child and Human Development

P.O. Box 571485
Washington, DC 20057
www.gucchdtacenter.georgetown.edu

Grant Information

www.grants.gov

Indian Health Service Division of Behavioral Health (IHS DBH)

Serves as the primary source of national advocacy, policy development, management and administration of behavioral health, alcohol and substance abuse, and family violence prevention programs for American Indian and Alaska Native people. Works in partnership with tribes and tribal organizations.

Institute of Behavioral Research—Community Treatment Forums

www.ibr.tcu.edu/pubs/datacoll/commtrt.html-ComTreatmentCosts

Journal of Rural Community Psychology

www.marshall.edu/jrcp
www.dbsalliance.org

The Kennedy Forum

124 Washington Street
Foxboro, MA 02035
www.thekennedyforum.org
www.paritytrack.org
www.onemind.org

Maine Rural Health Research Center

University of Southern Maine
Muskie School of Public Service
P.O. Box 9300
Portland, ME 04104-9300
207-780-4513
www.ruralhealthresearch.org/centers/maine

Mental Health America (MHA)

2000 N. Beauregard Street
6th Floor
Alexandria, VA 22311
Local: 703-864-7722
Toll-free: 800-969-6642
www.mentalhealthamerica.net

National Action Alliance for Suicide Prevention

The public/private partnership advancing the National Strategy for Suicide Prevention.
www.actionallianceforsuicideprevention.org/

National Alliance for the Mentally Ill (NAMI)

Colonial Place Three
2107 Wilson Blvd.
Suite 300
Arlington, VA 22201-3042
Local: 703-524-7600
Toll-free: 800-950-6264
www.nami.org

National Association for Rural Health (NARMH)

Works to develop and enhance rural mental health and substance abuse services, and to support mental health providers in rural areas.

25 Massachusetts Avenue NW
Suite 500
Washington, DC 20001
242-942-4276
info@narmh.org

National Center for Farmworker Health

1770 FM 967
Buda, TX 78610
www.ncfh.org

National Children's Center for Rural and Agricultural Health and Safety

www.marshfieldresearch.org

National Council for Behavioral Health

1400 K Street NW
Washington, DC 20005
www.thenationalcouncil.org

National Disaster Mental Health Training Program

National Center for Post-traumatic Stress Disorder
www.ptsd.va.gov/professional/ptsd-101.asp+/o

National Empowerment Center

599 Canal Street
Lawrence, MA 01840
978-685-1494
www.power2u.org

National Farm Medicine Center

Marshfield, WI
www.marshfieldresearch.org

National Institute of Mental Health (NIMH)

A biomedical and behavioral research agency that conducts research on mental and behavioral disorders and supports research on these topics in the United States. Some information available in Spanish.

Office of Rural Mental Health Research
6001 Executive Boulevard
Room 8184, MSC 9663
Bethesda, MD 20892-9663
Local: 301-443-4513
Toll-free: 866-615-6464
www.nimh.nih.gov

National Institute on Aging

Building 31 Center Dr., MSC 2292
Bethesda, MD 20892
800-222-2225
www.nia.nih.gov

National Mental Health Association (NMHA)

Each state has its own office.

2001 N. Beauregard Street
12th floor

Alexandria, VA 22311
Local: 703-684-7722
Toll-free: 800-433-5959
www.nmha.org

National Mental Health Consumer's Self-Help Clearinghouse

1211 Chestnut Street
Suite 1207
Philadelphia, PA 19107
215-636-6312
www.mhselfhelp.org

National Mental Health Information Center

P.O. Box 42557
Washington, DC 20015
800-789-2647
www.mentalhealth.samhsa.gov

National Organization of State Offices of Rural Health

www.nosorh.org

National Rural Behavioral Health Center (NRBHC)

Focuses on four components of rural behavioral health: rural disaster and trauma, violence prevention, occupational health, and health service delivery. Houses a team of behavioral health scientists, educators, scholars, and practitioners dedicated to improving the health care status of rural Americans.

National Rural Health Association

4501 College Blvd., #225
Leawood, KS 66211-1921
816-756-3140
www.ruralhealthweb.org

National Technical Assistance Center for Children's Mental Health

Georgetown University Center for Child and Human Development
P.O. Box 571485

Washington, DC 20057
www.gucchdtacenter.georgetown.edu

New York State Office of Rural Health

New York Department of Health Corning Tower
Room 1839
Empire State Plaza
Albany, NY 12237
518-402-0102
orh@health.state.ny.us

Office of Rural Health Policy (HRSA)

5600 Fishers Lane
Rockville, MD 20857
877-464-4772
www.hrsa.gov/ruralhealth

Office of Rural Mental Health Research (ORMHR)

National Institute of Mental Healthcare
6001 Executive Blvd.
Room 6200, MSC 9663
Bethesda, MD 20892-9663

President's New Freedom Commission on Mental Health

www.govinfo.library.unt.edu/mentalhealthcommission/reports

Rural Assistance Center

Rural Information Hub
School of Medicine and Health Sciences
Suite E231
1301 N. Columbia Road, Stop 9037
Grand Forks, ND 58202-1898
www.ruralhealthinfo.org

Rural Behavioral Health Organization

730 N. Franklin Street
Suite 501

Chicago, IL 60610-7224
Local: 312-642-0049
www.ruralbehavioralhealth.org

Rural Health Info

800-826-3632

Rural Health Information Hub

School of Medical and Health Sciences
Room 4520
501 N. Columbia Road
Stop 9037
Grand Forks, ND 58202-9037
800-270-1898
info@ruralhealthinfo.org

Rural Health Research Gateway

University of North Dakota Center for Rural Health
School of Medicine and Health Sciences
501 North Columbia Road, Stop 9037
Grand Forks, ND 58202-9037
info@ruralhealthresearch.org

Rural Information Center

USDA
10301 Battinure Avenue
Beltsville, MD 20705
www.nal.usda.gov

Rural People, Rural Policy

Institute for Emerging Issues
NC State University
Centennial Campus, Box 7406
Raleigh, NC 27695

Rural Policy Research Institute

Department of Health Management and Policy
University of Iowa College of Public Healthcare

145 N. Riverside Drive
Iowa City, IA 52242
www.rupri.org

Rural Psych

www.apa.org/practice/programs/rural

SAMHSA

Community Conversations About Mental Health Guide
www.mentalhealth.gov/talk/community-conversation
or www.samhsa.gov/community-conversations

SAMHSA Disaster Technical Assistance Center (DTAC)

Helps prepare states, territories, tribes, and local entities to deliver an effective mental health and substance misuse response to disasters.
www.mentalhealth.gov/dtac

SAMHSA's National Registry of Evidence-Based Programs and Practices

www.nrepp.samhsa.gov/ViewAll.aspx

South Central Mental Illness Research, Education and Clinical Center (MIRECC)

Focuses on equal access to quality mental health care for veterans in rural areas.
US Department of Veterans Affairs
Veteran's Crisis Line 800-273-8255
www.mirecc.va.gov

Substance Abuse and Mental Health Services Administration (SAMHSA)

Works to improve the quality and availability of prevention, treatment, and rehabilitative services in order to reduce illness, death, disability, and cost to society resulting from substance abuse and mental illnesses. Part of the US Department of Health and Human Services.
1 Choke Cherry Road

212 Mental Health Organizations

Rockville, MD 20857
877-726-4727
www.samhsa.gov

Substance Abuse Economics—RTI International

www.rti.org

Suicide Prevention Resource Center (SPRC)

Hotline phone: 800-273-TALK (8255), staffed 24/7.
www.sprc.org

Sustainable Communities Network

www.sustainable.org

Telemental Health Guide

University of Colorado
1250 14th Street
Denver, CO 80204
www.tmhguide.org

United States Department of Agriculture (USDA) Rural Development Office (National—states have offices as well)

1400 Independence Avenue SW
Room 5803, S STOP 3201
Washington, DC 20250–0506
www.rd.usda.org

United States Department of Agriculture (USDA)—Farm Service Agency

1400 Independence Avenue SW
STOP 0506
Washington, DC 20250–0506
www.fsa.usda.org

United States Department of Health and Human Services (HHS)

www.stopbullying.gov

Veterans Crisis Line

800-273-8255, press 1.

WICHE (Western Interstate Commission for Higher Education)

Mental Health Program
3035 Center Green Drive
Suite 200
Boulder, CO 80301-2204

W. K. Kellogg Foundation Evaluation Handbook

www.wkkf.org/knowledge-center/resources/

World Health Organization's European Headquarters

Avenue Appia 20
1202 Geneva
Switzerland
www.who.int

Recommended Reading

Agnew, Eleanor. (2004). *Back From the Land: How Young Americans Went to Nature in the 1970's and Why They Came Back*. Chicago: Ivan R. Dee.
Allen, R. L. (2002). *The American Farm Book*. Guilford, CT: The Lyons Press.
Bonta, Marcia, M. (1991). *Women in the Field: America's Pioneering Women Naturalists*. College Station: Texas A&M University Press.
Costa, Temra. (2010). *Farmer Jane: Women Changing the Way We Eat*. Layton, UT: Gibbs, Smith.
Ellison, Joan J. (1995). *Shepherdess: Notes from the Field*. West Lafayette, IN: Purdue University Press.
Emery, Carla. (2012). *Encyclopedia of Country Living, 40th Anniversary Edition*. North Adams, MA: Storey.
Fels, Tom. (2008). *Farm Friends: From the Late Sixties to the West Seventies and Beyond*. North Bennington, VT: Rural Science Institute.
Hewitt, Ben. (2009). *The Town That Food Saved*. Emmaus, PA: Rodale.
Ivanko, John and Kivirist, Lisa. (2004). *Rural Renaissance*. British Columbia: New Society.
Krupp, Ron. (2009). *Lifting the Yoke: Local Solutions to America's Farm and Food Crisis*. Montreal: Whetstone Books
Nearing, Helen and Nearing, Scott. (1989). *The Good Life*. New York: Schocken Books.
Old Farmer's Almanac. (2016). Dublin, NH: Yankee.
Perry, Michael. (2009). *Coop: A Year of Poultry, Pigs and Parenting*. New York: Harper Collins.
Schaper, Donna. (2007). *Grassroots Gardening: Rituals for Sustaining Activism*. New York: Avalon.
Solnit, Rebecca. (2009). *A Paradise Built in Hell*. New York: Viking.
Storey, John and Storey, Martha. (1999). *Basic Country Skills*. North Adams, MA: Storey.
Timmermeister, Kurt. (2011). *Growing a Farmer: How I Learned to Live Off the Land*. New York: W.W. Norton.
Timmermeister, Kurt. (2014). *Growing a Feast: The Chronicle of a Farm to Table Meal*. New York: W.W. Norton.
Ulrich, Laurel Thatcher. (2001). *The Age of Homespun—Objects and Stories in the Creation of an American Myth*. New York: Knopf.
Woginrich, Jenna. (2011). *Barnheart: The Incurable Longing for a Farm of One's Own*. North Adams, MA: Storey.
Woginrich, Jenna. (2013). *One Woman Farm*. Adams, MA: Storey.
Woginrich, Jenna. (2014). *Cold Antler Farm*. Boston: Shambhala Books.

Index

21st Century Cures Act 8, 21–23

AA (Alcoholics Anonymous) 149
AACP (American Association of Community Psychiatrists) 202
AAM (American Agriculture Movement) 176–178
AATA (American Art Therapy Association) 112–113
ACA (Affordable Care Act) 8, 12, 19–22, 32; implications of 20–21; need for affordable health insurance 85
acceptability 32–34
accessibility 29–30, 98
ACEs (adverse childhood experiences) 51, 136, 139–140
ADA (Americans with Disabilities Act) 70
addiction: heroin addiction 150–151; opioid epidemic 146–148; painkiller addiction 146–147; Substance Abuse and Mental Health Services Administration 17; *see also* alcohol abuse; substance abuse
ADHD (attention deficit hyperactivity disorder) 52, 105
Administration for Children & Families Office of Planning, Research and Evaluation 202
adolescents in rural America 55–56, 67, 113, 137; binge drinking 145; suicide rates 56
adoption of foster children 151–153
advocacy 189
affordability of treatment 34–38
AFSP (American Foundation for Suicide Prevention) 202
Agency for Healthcare Research and Quality 17
agricultural towns 3
agriculture: AAM 176–178; crop diversity 180; farm bill 81–83; farm crisis 78–79; rural farms 79; rural non-farms 79; statistics 179; sustainability 180
AHC (Accountable Health Communities) 193
AHR (Alliance for Health Reform) 183
Alaskan Natives in rural America 57–59; accessibility to mental health care 58–59; suicide rates 57–58
Albert, Eddie 49
alcohol abuse xvii, 45, 50, 58, 61, 68, 93, 116, 143, 145–147, 185, 190, 202; among adolescents 55; co-occurring disorders 144; DWI laws 145; FAS 58; prevention programs 146, 150; treatment methods 149
Alexander, Lamar 192
American Indians in rural America 57–59; accessibility to mental health care 58–59; suicide rates 57–58
American Journal of Public Health 36
antidepressants: SSRIs 11; tricyclics 9
anxiety 29; benzodiazepines 10; SSRIs 11
APA (American Psychiatric Association) 132; DSM 13
applying for grants 198
ARRA (American Recovery and Reinvestment Act) 105, 185
art therapists 112–113
As You Sow 176
Assistant Secretary for Mental Health 193
assisted-living facilities 56

216 *Index*

asylums 8; deinstitutionalization 9
availability of mental health practitioners 30–32

Back to the Land movement xviii, 175
barriers: logistical barriers to mental health 33; of rural residents to mental health services xiv, xvii–xviii, 28–29; to telepsychology 184–185
bartering for professional services 131
Beers, Clifford 9
behavioral health 5; tele-behavioral health 182–183; *see also* mental health
behavioral health aides 114
benzodiazepines 10
bill for the Construction of Mental Retardation Facilities and Community Health Centers 13
binge drinking 145
Binghamton Psychiatric Hospital 32
Bloom, Sandra 122–123
Blue Cross and Blue Shield 106
board of supervisors 44
bonding with nature 121–122
Botticelli, Michael 144
boundaries of clinical conversations 128
brain disorders 23
"brain drain" 66–67
BRAIN initiative 23
BRFSS (Behavioral Risk Factor Surveillance System) 62
Broken Heartland (Davidson) 78, 81–82
Bryan, William Jennings 83
Bush, George H.W. 8, 15
Bush, George W. 11, 18

CAIANH (Centers for American Indian and Alaska Native Health) 203
career paths for PNPs 109
carfentanil 148
Carter, Jimmy 8, 11, 14–15
Carter, Rosalynn 11, 14, 66, 82
case poverty 66
Catskills Mountains 178–179
CBT (cognitive behavioral therapy) 120–121, 124; -SP (cognitive behavioral therapy for suicide prevention) 160

CDC (Centers for Disease Control) 22; Evaluation Working Group 202
Center for Community-Based Children's Mental Health Research and Policy 124–125
Center for Rural Affairs 203
Center for Rural Entrepreneurship 55
Center for Rural Mental Health Studies 203
"central" schools 136
challenges in telepsychology 184–185
The Challenges of Rural Clinical Mental Health Counseling (Weigel) 129
Chambers, Alan 69
characteristics of successful mental health programs 197–198
Childhood Lost (Olfman) 52
children: ACEs 51–52, 139–140; ADHD 52; FAS 58; foster children 151–153; Joint Commission on the Mental Health of Children 10; mental health screening programs 139–140; National Children's Center for Rural and Agricultural Health and Safety 206; No Child Left Behind Act 194; parental incarceration 65; poor academic performance, causes of 137; post-disaster mental health interventions 95; regional schools 98–99; in rural America 51–53; Sanctuary Model 122–123; suicide rates in rural areas 158; victims of natural disasters 92–93
Christie, Chris 148
clients, responsibilities of in the therapy process 130
Clinton, Hillary Rodham 191, 194
Clinton Health Care Act 36
Clozaril 15
CMHC (Community Mental Health Centers) 46
CMS (Centers for Medicare and Medicaid Services) 203
CoCs (Continuums of Care) 72
collaboration 100; "National Counselor Licensure Endorsement Process" 197
collaborative care services 16–17
Commission on Mental Health 11
Committee on Rural Health and Human Services 63

A Common Struggle (Kennedy) 14
Community Mental Health Centers 13; Act of 1963 45; collaborative care services 16–17; limited access to care 30
community psychology 123–124
Community Services Board 13, 45, 46
"comorbid" diagnoses 25
competition in mental health field 32
Comprehensive Behavioral Health Reform and Recovery Act 192
confidentiality, HIPAA 184
CONTAC (Consumer Organization and Networking Technical Assistance Center) 203
continuing education 129–130
co-occurring disorders 144, 147–148
Cooperative Extension 80–81, 92
Corrections and Mental Health Collaboration Act 23
counseling: boundaries of clinical conversations 128; characteristics of successful mental health programs 197–198; crisis counseling 92; Family Support Group Program 49; Gestalt therapy 93; grief counseling 183; itinerant counseling 115–116; LCSWs 110–111; licensed mental health counselors 110; Mental Health First Aid 191; "National Counselor Licensure Endorsement Process" 197; pastoral counselors 115; peer advocates 113–115; post-disaster mental health interventions 95; professional counseling practice 110; rural counseling programs 44; school counseling 93; spiritual beliefs 94; for suicidal individuals 159–161; telepsychology 183
counterculture 121
Credentialed Family Peer Advocates 114
crisis counseling 92; mobile crisis teams 111–112; schools 93
crisis respite 111–112
Critical Access Hospitals xviii
Critical Rural Theory 3, 174–175
crop diversity 180
CSB (Community Services Board) 13, 45–46
culture of rural living 48; adolescents 55–56; American Indians 57–59; disabled individuals 70–71; elderly 56; families 49; homelessness 71–73; incarcerated populations 64–65; infants and children 51–53; LGBTQ 68–70; men 49–50; poverty 66–67; refugees and undocumented immigrants 60–61; sex offenders 64–65; veterans 59–60; victims of domestic violence 62–64; weapons ownership 67–68; women 50–51
Cures Act of 2016 22–23, 148

dance/movement therapy 112–113
Davidson, Osha Grey 77–78, 81–82
Decade of the Brain 8, 15
decarceration 188, 189
deciding to enter private practice 168–170
defining: frontier 3–4; rural areas 2–4
deinstitutionalization 9; in Delaware County, New York 31–32; IMD 10; OBRA 11; "snake pits" 14; Willowbrook 10
Delaware County, New York xvi, 1; deinstitutionalization in 31–32; statistics 4–5
Department of Housing and Urban Development, CoCs 72
Department of Veterans Affairs 17
depopulation of rural areas 99
depression 29; among rural American women 50–51; pre- and post-partum depression 50; and suicide 157; treatment 9
director of community mental health services 45
disabilities: case poverty 66; intellectually disabled individuals in rural America 70–71; physically disabled individuals in rural America 70
disasters: man-made disasters 95–96; mobile crisis teams 111–112; natural disasters 91–95; phases of 94
"disconnected youth" 55
Dix, Dorothea 9
Dorgan, Byron 17
drama therapy 112–113
Dreamland 148
drinking: among adolescents 55; among American Indian youth 58; *see also* alcohol abuse

drug abuse xvii, 61, 64, 65, 69, 71, 93, 116, 143, 185, 144–145; among adolescents 55; co-occurring disorders 144; deaths occurring from 21, 55, 143; heroin addiction 150–151; methamphetamine abuse 144–145; morphine 148–149; National Survey on Drug Use and Health 22; opioid epidemic 146–148; prevention programs 150; treatment methods 149–150
Drug Abuse Treatment Cost Analysis Program 204
DSM (*Diagnostic and Statistical Manual of Mental Disorders*) 13, 36
DV (domestic violence) xviii, 62–64, 80, 122, 139, 150, 152, 158, 185
DWI (driving while intoxicated) laws 145

Early Start 52
Eastern Tennessee State University Department of Psychology 204
EBPs (evidence-based programs) 193
eco-guardianship 122
"economic gardening" 180
Economic Research Service 3; (USDA) 2
ecopsychology 121–122
education: "central" schools 136; characteristics of successful mental health programs 197–198; continuing education 129–130; emotional literacy education 138; internships for rural health graduate programs 176; MSW 110–111; poor academic performance, causes of 137; regional schools 98–99; *see also* schools
Eisenhower, Dwight D. 83
elderly in rural America 56; suicide rates in rural areas 158; victims of natural disasters 93–94
"emotional haze" 139
emotional literacy education 138; as treatment for suicidality 160
Endangered Spaces, Enduring Places 178
entrepreneurship in the rural economy 174–175
ethics in rural mental health 127–129
Executive Order #13575 37

families in rural America 49
family farming 87

Family Support Group Program 49
family support specialists 188
family therapists 110
Family-to-Family 49
famous farming quotes 83
Farm Beginnings program 36
farm bill 81–83; food stamps 82
farm crisis 78, 79; *Broken Heartland* (Davidson) 77–78, 80–82; personalizing 85–87; social isolation of farmers 80; suicide rates during 80
Farm Policy Facts 204
Farm Service Agency 35
farm subsidy program 35–36
farming 48; agricultural policy 176–177; Cooperative Extension 80–81; family farming 87; famous quotes 83; fatalities caused by 79; industrialized 175; industrialized farming 180; right-to-farm laws 82–83; and rural economy 174–175; statistics 84, 179
FAS (fetal alcohol syndrome) 58
fatalism 61–62
fatalities: caused by alcohol abuse 145; caused by farming accidents 79
Federal Office of Rural Health Policy 52; "disconnected youth" 55
federal rural programs, farm subsidy program 35–36
FedStats 204
Fetal Alcohol Syndrome 51–53, 58
fentanyl 148
firearms: fatalities from suicide in rural areas 156; weapons ownership in rural America 67–68
floods, hundred-year floods 91
food stamps 82
foster children 151–153
four A's and an S: acceptability 32–34; accessibility 29–30; affordability 34–38; availability 30–32; stigma 38–39
fracking 95
Francis, Richard 53
frontier, defining 3–4
Frontier Mental Health Services Resource Network 204

Gabor, Eva 49
Galbraith, John Kenneth 66
Gay, Lesbian, and Straight Educational Network 204

geographic accessibility 30
Georgetown University Center for Child and Human Development 204
Gestalt therapy 93
ghettoization 81
"ghost sickness" 57
GLSEN (Gay, Lesbian, and Straight Educational Network) 69
goals of President's New Freedom Commission on Mental Health 18
Goldschmidt, Walter 176
gossip 6, 131, 169
Graham, Lindsay 18
grants: applying for 198; Morrill Land Grant Act of 1862 81; Rural Renaissance Act 18; state grants 198
Green Acres 49
Greene, Gene 192–193
"greening up" 178
grief counseling 183
groundwater contamination 179
group therapy 196
guns: fatalities from suicide in rural areas 156; weapons ownership in rural America 67–68

Harrington, Michael 66, 175
Harrison Act of 1914 149
Head Start 51
health insurance: ACA 12, 19–22; Blue Cross and Blue Shield 106; HIPAA 33, 182, 192; need for 85; reimbursement policies 106; Wellstone-Domenici Mental Health Parity and Addiction Equity Act 12
health professional shortage area (HPSA) 32, 105, 182
Health Resources and Services Administration 15, 17
"heartbreak syndrome" 57
heroin 37, 61, 144, 146–148, 150, 161
heroin addiction 150–151
HHS (US Department of Health and Human Services) 2, 20, 213; Opioid Initiative 146; ORP 2
HIPAA (Health Insurance Portability and Accountability Act) 33, 182, 192; confidentiality 184
Hippocrates 8
history of rural mental health 8–18
HITECH (Health Information Technology for Economic and Clinical Health) Act 192

homelessness 14, 58, 71–73, 139, 183
Homestead Act 99
homosexuality, LGBTQ in rural America 68–70
hospitals: Binghamton Psychiatric Hospital 32; collaborative care services 16–17; Community Mental Health Centers 13; Critical Access Hospitals xviii; deinstitutionalization 9; telepsychology 183
Housing First model 71–72
H.R. 34 22–23
HRSA (Health Resources and Services Administration) 105
hundred-year floods 91
hurricanes: Irene 91; Sandy 96

IHS DBH (Indian Health Service Division of Behavioral Health) 205
IMD (Institutions for Mental Diseases) 8, 10, 14, 191
immigration: migrant workers in rural America 61–62; undocumented immigrants in rural America 60–61
implications: of ACA 20–21; of Medicaid redesign 23–24
improving rural mental health services 192–197
incarcerated populations in rural America 64–65
industrialized farming 175, 180
infants in rural America 51–53; FAS 58
information networks 190
innovation 3–4; technophobia 184–185; telepsychology 182–183
Institute of Behavioral Research—Community Treatment Forums 205
insular poverty 66
insurance: ACA 12, 19–22; 85, 114; Blue Cross and Blue Shield 106; HIPAA 33, 182, 192; reimbursement policies 106, 110, 194; laws xiv, xvi, 11, 16, 18, 116; Wellstone-Domenici Mental Health Parity and Addiction Equity Act 12
intellectually disabled individuals in rural America 70–71
International Congress on Mental Hygiene 9
internships for rural health graduate programs 176
interventions: characteristics of successful mental health programs

220 *Index*

197–198; Mental Health First
Aid 191
itinerant counseling 115–116

Johnson, Lyndon B. 10
Joint Commission on Mental Illness
and Mental Health 12
Joint Commission on the Mental
Health of Children 10
*Journal of Rural Community
Psychology* 136–137, 205

Kellogg Foundation 35–36
Kennedy, John F. 10, 12, 83; "Special
Message to the Congress on Mental
Illness and Mental Retardation"
12–13
Kennedy, Patrick xiii, 10, 14, 15, 19,
36, 64, 137, 148, 191
Kennedy, Robert 10
Kennedy, Rosemary 13
Kennedy, Ted 14, 137
Kennedy Forum 18, 71, 137, 139,
205

land grants, Morrill Land Grant Act of
1862 81
Land Stewardship Project 36
*Last Child in the Woods: Saving Our
Children From Nature-Deficit
Disorder* (Louv) 121
Latin Americans in rural America
61–62
LCATs (Licensed Creative Arts
Therapists) 34
LCSWs (licensed clinical social
workers) 110–111
legislation: *21st Century Cures
Act* 8, 21–22; ACA 8, 12; ADA
70; bill for the Construction of
Mental Retardation Facilities and
Community Health Centers 13;
Community Mental Health Centers
Act of 1963 45; Corrections and
Mental Health Collaboration Act
23; Cures Act of 2016 22–23;
farm bill 81–83; Homestead Act
99; Maternal and Child Health
and Mental Retardation Planning
Amendment 10; Medicare
Telehealth Parity Act of 2014
20–21; *Mental Health Parity Act
of 2008* 8, 18–19; National Mental
Health Act 9; New Homestead
Act 36; No Child Left Behind Act
194; OBRA 11; right-to-farm laws
82–83; Rural Renaissance Act 36;
Wellstone-Domenici Mental Health
Parity and Addiction Equity Act 12,
193
LGBTQ in rural America 68–70
Libous, Tom 31
license portability 21, 185, 197
licensed marriage and family therapists
110
licensed mental health counselors 110
licensing, psychologists 108–109
licensure laws 106; in New Hampshire
189
limited access to care 30
loans, Rural Renaissance Act 18
local government: CMHC 46; CSB
45–46; structure of 44–45
logistical barriers to mental health 33
Louv, Richard 121

Maine Rural Health Research Center
205; study 145–146
Manderscheid, Ron 19–20, 38, 39,
64, 71, 114, 148, 192, 194
man-made disasters 95–96
marriage: licensed marriage and family
therapists 110; serial monogamy in
rural areas 98
Maternal and Child Health and Mental
Retardation Planning Amendment
10
Medicaid 10, 19–21, 56, 110; IMD
14; redesign, implications of 23–24
Medicare 10, 105; reimbursement
rates 34–35; Telehealth Parity Act of
2014 20–21
Memorial Day parade 40–41
men in rural America 49–50; suicide
among 157
mental health 5; advocacy 189;
affordability of treatment 34–38;
asylums 8; barriers to treatment
28–29; characteristics of successful
mental health programs 197–198;
collaborative care services
16–17; community approach
to 137; Corrections and Mental
Health Collaboration Act 23;
deinstitutionalization 9; DSM
13; ethics in rural mental health

127–129; history of rural mental health 8–18; improving rural mental health services 192–197; infant mental health 51; interventions 188; Joint Commission on Mental Illness and Mental Health 12; limited access to care 30; NAMI 11; NARMH 33–34; National Mental Health Act 9; New Freedom Commission on Mental Health 15–17; NIMH 9; performance standards 17; post-disaster mental health interventions 95; public health approach to 124–125; rural counseling programs 44; school-based screening programs 139–140; screening 191; "Special Message to the Congress on Mental Illness and Mental Retardation" 12–13; statistics on rural mental health 24–25; Surgeon General's report on 19; timeline of mental health in rural America 9–12; *see also* mental health practitioners
Mental Health America 9, 114, 190, 205
Mental Health First Aid 191
Mental Health Parity Act of 2008 8, 11–12, 18–19
mental health practitioners: art therapists 112–113; challenges in telepsychology 184–185; competition among 32; continuing education 129–130; a day in the life of 165–168; deciding to enter private practice 168–170; family support specialists 188; itinerant counseling 115–116; LCSWs 110–111; licensed marriage and family therapists 110; licensed mental health counselors 110; licensure laws 106, 189; mobile crisis teams 111–112; pastoral counselors 115; PCPs 115; peer advocates 113–115; PNPs 109; primary care providers 105; psychiatrists 108; psychologists 108–109; referral systems 31; in rural areas 5–6; scope of practice 105–108; training 17; training for rural work 116–117; turf wars 104–107
Mental Health Professional Practice Act 107
Mental Health Systems Act 11

mental illness: co-occurring disorders 144; and poverty 97; and suicide 157–158
Mentally Ill Offender Community Transition Program 64
methamphetamine abuse 144–145
A Mind That Found Itself (Beers) 9
mobile crisis teams 111–112
monoamine oxidase inhibitors 9
morphine 148–149
Morrill Land Grant Act of 1862 81
MSW (master's degree in social work) 110–111
multiculturalism 1
mu-opioid receptors 148
music therapy 112–113
Muskie School of Public Service report 105, 107

NA (Narcotics Anonymous) 149
NACBHDD (National Association of County Behavioral Health & Developmental Disability Directors) 19–20, 38, 64–65, 115
NACMH (National Advisory Council on Migrant Health) 61–62
naloxone 146, 148
NAMI (National Alliance for the Mentally Ill) 11, 23, 206; Credentialed Family Peer Advocates 114; Family-to-Family 49
NARMH (National Association for Rural Mental Health) 33–34, 194, 206
National Advisory Committee on Rural Health and Human Services 51
National Alliance to End Homelessness 72–73
National Center for Farmworker Health 206
National Certified Peer Specialist 114
National Children's Center for Rural and Agricultural Health and Safety 206
National Conference on Mental Health 12
National Council for Behavioral Health 206
"National Counselor Licensure Endorsement Process" 197
National Disaster Mental Health Training Program 207

National Empowerment Center 207
National Farm Medicine Center 207
National Health Service Corps scholarship 192
National Institute on Aging 207
National Mental Health Act 9
National Mental Health Consumer's Self-Help Clearinghouse 208
National Mental Health Information Center 208
National Organization of State Offices of Rural Health 208
National Rural Health Association 188, 208
National Rural Mental Health Advisory Committee 15
National Survey on Drug Use and Health 22
National Technical Assistance Center for Children's Mental Health 208
Native Americans in rural America: suicide rates 57–58; suicide rates among 157, 158
natural disasters 91–95; children as victims of 92–93; crisis counseling 92; elderly as victims of 93–94; planning for 91–92
"natural" towns 3
Nature and Madness (Shepherd) 122
need for affordable health insurance 85
needs assessments in rural areas 99–100
nervios 61
New Deal 12
new federalism 11
New Freedom Commission on Mental Health 15–17
New Hampshire, mental health licensure laws 189
New Homestead Act 17–18, 36
New Mexico 108–109
New York State Coalition Against Domestic Violence 63–64
New York State Office of Rural Health 209
NHSC (National Health Services Corporation) 105
NIH (National Institutes of Health) 15
NIMH (National Institute of Mental Health) 9, 17, 207
No Child Left Behind Act 194
"non-metropolitan" areas 2
NRBHC (National Rural Behavioral Health Center) 208

nurses, PNPs 31 *see also* Psychiatric Nurse Practitioners

Obama, Barack 12, 37, 144; ACA 19–22
Obamacare 24, 69, 185, 194
OBRA (Omnibus Budget Reconciliation Act) 11
obstacles to mental health treatment, accessibility 29–30
Olfman, Sharna 52–53
OMB (Office of Management and Budget), defining rural 2
omnibus 81
opioids 61, 143, 144, 146, 150
opioid epidemic 143, 146–148
Opioid Initiative 146
ORMHR (Office of Rural Mental Health Research) 209
ORP (Office of Rural Health Policy) 2, 15
outreach 115–116
OxyContin 143

Pacely, Megan 68
painkillers, addiction to 146–147
parental incarceration 65
parity 14, 22, 36, 37, 146, 148, 159, 193, 194; Medicare Telehealth Parity Act of 2014 20–21; *Mental Health Parity Act of 2008* 8, 11, 12, 18–19; reducing stigmatization 38–39; Wellstone-Domenici Mental Health Parity and Addiction Equity Act 12, 13, 193
participation, reducing stigmatization 39
pastoral counselors 115
Paxil 11
payment, bartering for professional services 131
PCPs *See* primary care physicians
PDR (Physicians' Desk Reference) 3
peer advocates 113–115, 189
peers, reducing stigmatization 39
performance standards for mental healthcare 17
persistent poverty 180
phases of disasters 94
physical health 5
physically disabled individuals in rural America 70
planning: for natural disasters 91–92; Strategic Prevention Framework 100

PNPs (*see* psychiatric nurse practitioners) 31, 109
policy: agricultural policy 176–177; Federal Office of Rural Health Policy 52; omnibus 81; rural policy 37–38
poor academic performance, causes of 137
post-disaster mental health interventions 95
poverty 66–67, 97; depopulation of rural areas 99; homelessness 71–73; needs assessments in rural areas 99–100; persistent poverty 180; statistics 97
practice: deciding to enter private practice 168–170; reducing stigmatization 38–39
pre- and post-partum depression 50
prescription drugs: carfentanil 148; Clozaril 15; fentanyl 148; naloxone 146; OxyContin 143; painkiller addiction 146–147; Prozac 15; psychotropic drugs 108, 115; SSRIs 11; Thorazine 9; Village Drug Reference 3
Presidential Commission on Mental Health/ President's Commission on Mental Health 14–15, 192
President's New Freedom Commission on Mental Health 8, 11, 15, 136, 188; goals 18; recommendations 15–17, 140, 190
prevalence of suicide in rural areas 156–158
prevention of suicide 158–159
primary care physicians 115
primary care providers 16, 19, 22, 30–35, 63, 105, 106, 108–109, 115, 124, 140, 157, 188, 192
privacy in rural areas 168
private practice, deciding to enter 168–170
professional counseling practice 110
The Professional Counselor (Imig) 128
promotion, reducing stigmatization 38–39
Prozac 11, 15
Psychiatric Nurse Practitioners (PNPs). 31, 109
psychiatrists 108
psychologists 108–109; challenges in telepsychology 184–185; community psychology 123–124; ecopsychology 121–122; telepsychology 182–183
psychotherapy 120
psychotropic drugs, prescribing 108, 115
PTSD (post-traumatic stress disorder) 59–60, 90
public health approach to mental health 124–125

Quinones, Sam 148, 149

Reagan, Ronald 11
recommendations: characteristics of successful mental health programs 197–198; for expanding mental health service availability 52; improving rural mental health services 192–197; Muskie School of Public Service report 107; of NARMH 34; in New Freedom Commission on Mental Health 15–17; President's New Freedom Commission on Mental Health 140, 190
recovery from suicidality 161
recreation centers in rural communities 190
redesign of Medicaid, implications of 23–24
reducing stigmatization 38–39
referral systems 31
refugees in rural America 60–61
regional schools 98–99
reimbursement rates, Medicare 34–35
relationships in rural areas 130–131; and suicide 158–159
religion: pastoral counselors 115; spiritual beliefs 94; *see also* treatment philosophies
renewable energy 178
research in rural and frontier areas 191
right-to-farm laws 82–83
risk factors for suicide 158–159
Rivera, Geraldo 10
Roosevelt, Franklin D. 9; New Deal 12
Roszak, Theodore 121
Roxbury, New York xvii
rural areas 1–2; deciding to enter private practice in 168–170; defining 2–4; depopulation of 99; gossip 6; groundwater contamination 179; history of rural mental health 8–18; mental

224   Index

health professionals 5–6; needs
   assessments in 99–100; New
   Homestead Act 17–18; poverty
   97, 98; privacy in 168; recreation
   centers 190; relationships in
   130–131; serial monogamy in 98;
   statistics on rural mental health
   24–25; substance abuse in 147;
   timeline of mental health in rural
   America 9–12; topography 4;
   weather 4; *see also* culture of rural
   living; frontier
Rural Assistance Center 209
Rural Behavioral Health Care 28
Rural Behavioral Health Organization
   209
Rural Behavioral Health Programs
   and Promising Practices 193; Guide
   197–198
rural counseling programs 44
rural decay 98
rural economy 174–180; agriculture
   176–178; "economic gardening"
   180; entrepreneurship 174–175;
   farming 174–175; supermarkets
   174; tourism 175–176
rural farms 79
Rural Health Information Hub 100,
   210
Rural Health Research Gateway 210
Rural Information Center 210
Rural Mental Health 56
*Rural Mental Health and Psychological
   Treatment: A Review for
   Practitioners* 98
rural non-farms 79
Rural Policy Research Institute 210
Rural Renaissance Act 18, 36
rural residents, barriers to mental
   health services xiv, xvii–xviii
Rural Subcommittee 30, 31, 190, 193
Rust Belt 98

SAMHSA (Substance Abuse
   and Mental Health Services
   Administration) 22–23, 97, 114,
   211–212; Strategic Prevention
   Framework 100; website 100
Sanctuary Model 122–123
schizophrenia 15
school bus environment 136–137
schools: alcohol abuse prevention
   145–146; "central" schools 136;
   consolidation 137; crisis counseling
   93; mental health screening

programs 139–140; regional schools
   98–99; rural schools, housing
   mental health programs in 138;
   telepsychology 183
*The Science and Pseudoscience of
   Children's Mental Health* (Olfman) 53
scope of practice 105–108; art
   therapists 112–113; LCSWs
   110–111; licensed marriage and
   family therapists 110; licensed
   mental health counselors 110;
   mobile crisis teams 111–112;
   pastoral counselors 115; PCPs 115;
   peer advocates 113–115; PNPs
   109; psychiatrists 108; psychologists
   108–109
SEDs (serious emotional disturbances)
   44
Seeking Safety 122–123
S.E.L.F. tool 123
self-poisoning 156
self-reliance 6, 169
self-stigma 38
serial monogamy in rural areas 98
serotonin, SSRIs 11, 15
sex offenders in rural America 64–65
sexual orientation, LGBTQ in rural
   America 68–70
Shepherd, Paul 122
"snake pits" 14
SNAP (Supplemental Nutrition
   Assistance Program) 82
social isolation of farmers 80
social workers 110–111, 151–153
"Special Message to the Congress
   on Mental Illness and Mental
   Retardation" 12–13
spiritual beliefs 94
SPOA (Single Point of Access)
   program 168
SPRC (Suicide Prevention Resource
   Center) 212
SSRIs (selective serotonin reuptake
   inhibitors) 11, 15
state grants 198
statistics: on farming 84, 179; on
   LGBTQ students in rural America
   69–70; on poverty 97; regarding
   Delaware County, New York 4–5;
   on rural mental health 24–25; on
   suicide 157
The Stepping Up Initiative 65
stereotypes 38
stigma 38–39; and acceptability
   32–34; as barrier to mental health

treatment 28; self-stigma 38; of suicidality 159
Strategic Prevention Framework 97, 100
stress, PTSD 59–60
structure of local government 44–45
substance abuse 144–145; alcohol abuse 145–146; among adolescents 55; among rural residents 147; co-occurring disorders 144, 147–148; heroin addiction 150–151; methamphetamine abuse 144–145; morphine 148–149; opioid epidemic 146–148; prevention programs 150; treatment methods 149–150
Substance Abuse and Mental Health Services Administration 17
suicide 161–162; AFSP 202; among American Indians and Alaskan Natives 57–58; among farmers 79, 80; among rural adolescents 56; among the elderly 56; CBT-SP 160; and emotional literacy education 160; gun deaths 156; monetary cost of 157–158; prevalence of in rural areas 156–158; preventing 158–161; recovery from suicidality 161; risk factors 158–159; self-poisoning 156; statistics 157; treatment for suicidality 159–161
supermarkets 174
Surgeon General's report on mental health 19
surveys, National Survey on Drug Use and Health 22
The Survival of Rural America (Wood) 35, 99
sustainability of school-based mental health programs 139
Sustainable Communities Network 212
susto 61
Swift, Jonathon 83
symptoms of fentanyl exposure 148

TBI (traumatic brain injury) 23
technical assistance programs 17
technophobia 184–185
tele-behavioral health 182–183
telehealth, Medicare Telehealth Parity Act of 2014 20–21
telemedicine 12, 18, 21, 32, 52, 185
Telemental Health Guide 212

telepsychology 182–183; challenges in 184–185
therapy 195; art therapists 112–113; CBT 120–121; client responsibilities in the therapy process 130; Gestalt therapy 93; group therapy 196; psychotherapy 120; recovery from suicidality 161; telepsychology 185; trauma-informed 124
Thorazine 9
timeline of mental health in rural America 9–12
topography of rural areas 4
tourism and the rural economy 175–176, 180
town supervisor 44, 45
towns 99; agricultural 3; board of supervisors 44; CMHC 46; CSB 45–46; director of community mental health services 45; "natural" 3; structure of local government 44–45
training: continuing education 129–130; licensed marriage and family therapists 110; of mental health practitioners 17; National Disaster Mental Health Training Program 207; for rural work 116–117
trauma: ACEs 139–140; PTSD 90
trauma-informed therapy 124
treatment: accessibility 29–30; affordability 34–38; barriers of rural residents to mental health services 28–29; for depression 9; Family Support Group Program 49; for PTSD 59–60; for suicidal individuals 159–161; *see also* treatment philosophies
treatment philosophies: CBT 120–121; community psychology 123–124; ecopsychology 121–122; public health approach to mental health 124–125; Sanctuary Model 122–123; trauma-informed therapy 124
tricyclics 9
Truman, Harry S. 9
Trump, Donald 148
turf wars between practitioner categories 106–107

undocumented immigrants in rural America 60–61
universities, internships for rural health graduate programs 176

unsolicited information, filtering 128–129
urban-centric point of view 1, 3
urbanormativity xiv, 1, 179
US Census Bureau 2; 2000 census 4
US Office of Rural Health Policy 2
USDA (US Department of Agriculture) 35, 212; Economic Research Service 2–3; farm subsidy program 35–36

VA (Veterans Administration) 59
Veterans Crisis Line 213
veterans in rural America 12, 16, 17, 23, 59–60, 65, 71, 113
victims of domestic violence in rural America 62–64
victims of natural disasters: children 92–93; elderly 93–94
Village Drug Reference 3
violence, weapons ownership in rural America 67–68

W. K. Kellogg Foundation Evaluation Handbook 213
Washington, George 83
weapons ownership in rural America 50, 67–68
weather: natural disasters 91–95; in rural areas 4
websites: CDC Evaluation Working Group 202; Center for Rural Affairs 203; Center for Rural Mental Health Studies 203; Drug Abuse Treatment Cost Analysis Program 204; Eastern Tennessee State University Department of Psychology 204; Farm Policy Facts 204; FedStats 204; Frontier Mental Health Services Resource Network 204; Gay, Lesbian, and Straight Educational Network 204; Georgetown University Center for Child and Human Development 204; grants.gov 198; Journal of Rural Community Psychology 205; Kennedy Forum 205; Maine Rural Health Research Center 205; Mental Health America 205; Mental Health First Aid 191; NAMI 206; NARMH 206; National Center for Farmworker Health 206; National Children's Center for Rural and Agricultural Health and Safety 206; National Council for Behavioral Health 206; National Disaster Mental Health Training Program 207; National Empowerment Center 207; National Farm Medicine Center 207; National Institute on Aging 207; National Mental Health Consumer's Self-Help Clearinghouse 208; National Mental Health Information Center 208; National Organization of State Offices of Rural Health 208; National Rural Health Association 208; National Technical Assistance Center for Children's Mental Health 209; New York State Office of Rural Health 209; NIMH 207; Rural Assistance Center 209; Rural Behavioral Health Organization 210; Rural Health Information Hub 100, 210; Rural Health Research Gateway 210; Rural Policy Research Institute 211; SAMHSA 100, 211; SPRC 212; Sustainable Communities Network 212; Telemental Health Guide 212
Weigel, Daniel 129
Wellstone-Domenici Mental Health Parity and Addiction Equity Act 12, 193
White House Office of National Drug Control Policy 144
White House Rural Council 37
WHO (World Health Organization) 13, 125, 213
WICHE (Western Interstate Commission for Higher Education) 213
Willowbrook mental health facility 10
Wilson, E.O. 121
Within Our Reach 66
women in rural America 50–51; DV 62–64; suicide among 157

Zoloft 11

Made in United States
Orlando, FL
14 May 2023